THE MODERN GUIDE TO SKIN CARE AND BEAUTY

by Irwin I. Lubowe, M.D., F.A.C.A.
with Harry L. Ober

Illustrated

London
George Allen & Unwin Ltd
Ruskin House   Museum Street

The distribution or mention of this book by any commercial
organization does not constitute endorsement by the author.

First published in Great Britain in 1975

ISBN 0 04 616015 9

Grateful acknowledgment is made to Ar-Ex Products Company and to
Hairdo and Beauty magazine, in whose December, 1972, issue it appeared,
for permission to reprint the chart in Appendix I; to Health Research for
the chart in Appendix II; to Faberge, Inc., for the photographs, except
where other credit is specified; and to *Today's Health*, published by the
American Medical Association, for the diagrams on pages 24 and 109.

Printed in Great Britain by
William Clowes & Sons, Limited
London, Beccles and Colchester

To my wife, Ruth, whose love, cooperation and
personal sacrifices have made this book possible

Contents

List of Illustrations

Preface

The basis for a new book should be new ideas. The basis for this one is, I believe, many new ideas whose time has come.

When the author's *New Hope for Your Skin* was published in 1965, it was by design a comprehensive summary of the most significant advances in the science of dermatology up till then. It also suggested a number of areas in which further breakthroughs appeared imminent—and "imminent" in terms of science may mean as much as a decade.

The original book was revised several times to include new developments that appeared to have lasting value, and each edition was well received. But over the eight years since its first publication, *New Hope for Your Skin* has reached the limit of reasonable architectural expansion. Adding more wings, ells, and extensions would not be a practicable solution for accommodating the new knowledge that has accumulated. A wholly new structure is indicated, some of its divisions smaller and some larger, according to changes in emphasis now required.

The reasons for a new book at this time are as compelling as they are interesting. While medicine formerly held itself largely apart from other sciences not immediately concerned with physical or mental diseases, such aloofness is no longer possible. Medical science has had to recognize that it must adjust to and make provision for new problems arising from our era's radical changes in life styles.

Some of these problems used to crop up occasionally but remained statistically too insignificant to attract major attention. Now, however, shifts in human behavior have suddenly made these problems more common and medical science has responded by finding new solutions.

In America's puritanical society of the nineteenth century, for example, skins were as vulnerable to chemical cosmetics as they are today. But "cosmetic skin" was an unknown problem for the simple reason that almost nobody used chemical cosmetics. Since 1960 there has been a massive proliferation of new cosmetic products and a consequent surge in skin and other body reactions to them. These are seldom due to impure chemicals but rather to the fact that the broader use of chemical cosmetics triggers allergic explosions among potentially susceptible users. The casualty list is further enlarged by men, who now make common use of one kind of cosmetic or another. At the root, then, was not a new medical problem but a new social development.

Yet cosmetics are not a major dermatological problem. Other social changes have brought with them far more skin abnormalities. What else has happened since 1960 or so? Young people, apparently reacting to new levels of emotional tension, are coming up with a startling increase in acne, which is clearly associated with emotional turbulence. To aggravate matters, long hair styles—which demand the most meticulous hygiene—are making disorders of the skin and hair even more difficult to control. Worse, the faddish use of marijuana and more powerful drugs has come under rising suspicion as another skin and hair troublemaker.

But even the most prudent and sensible—qualities that were once fair assurance of a clear skin as well as conscience—are exposed today to new onslaughts upon their skin. The thickening of urban air pollution has brought about a virtual epidemic of what I have called "City Skin," a condition to which no city dweller has a natural immunity. Consider its gravity in terms of the historical population shift of the sixties, when the majority of Americans were for the first time centered in cities rather than in rural areas.

The sixties also witnessed a massive spread of the use of the Pill, the first contraceptive for which total effectiveness could reasonably be claimed. Apart from other suspicions about its consequences that have prompted serious controversy, there is no question that its prolonged use has resulted in a serious skin problem among *some* women.

The past decade has also seen a continued shaving of hours from the average work week—a trend in which a four-day week is now contemplated. This translates for many people into more hours in the sun, and thus more skin damage, more permanent freckling, and surely more skin cancer. Longer vacation periods and increased traveling also add up to more holidays in tropical or semi-tropical climates and other more distant and alien environments. The still greater amount of time being spent on wintry ski slopes presents fresh skin hazards.

Perhaps the most vexing of the new problems spring, paradoxically, from the continuing extension of our average life expectancy. The other side of that coin is that the lot of the aging man and woman is becoming ever more distressing as our society gives rising emphasis to the value of being young, young, young, sharpening the frustration of the elderly about being old, old, old. Though they know that the difference is in many respects more apparent than real, they also know that a young-appearing skin can be a most convincing equalizer. To the extent that the aging of the skin can be reversed—or arrested—many people naturally go to considerable lengths to achieve it, and they are now finding dermatologists who are both sympathetic and capable.

These, then, are among the reasons for a new book at this time. It is designed for all who have skin problems they would like to know more about, who want to know how to recognize a problem early enough to turn it aside easily, or who seek guidance on how to avoid future problems.

For readers concerned about the effects of advancing seniority on the skin, I shall offer some advice on how to hold back the marks of time as long as possible.

In gathering material for this book during many years of specialized practice, I have read many scientific journals and magazines. I have consulted with cosmetic chemists, beauty counselors, and editors of beauty magazines as well as dermatological and other medical authorities. Translation of complex scientific data into laymen's language will, of course, sometimes result in a reduced degree of descriptive accuracy, adequate for the general reader but unsatisfactory to the scientist who works in precise terminology. It is not my purpose to provide a "do-it-yourself manual" for the treatment of skin diseases that may require medical attention. The common dermatological disorders are briefly discussed in Chapter 10.

My hope is that the book will be helpful to readers in all of the groups mentioned above, and that it may also prove useful as a general reference source for anyone seeking information about the skin.

New York, 1973

I. I. L.

THE MODERN
GUIDE TO
SKIN CARE
AND BEAUTY

1

Your Skin: What It Is – and Does

The skin, big as life and uniquely shaped, is not only one of the more complex organs of the body but also the largest one, measuring, in the average person, about eighteen square feet. It works harder than the others and is no one-function specialist. In structure it is composed of a number of closely connected layers, with sublayers having distinct identities. The three layers are:

1. The *epidermis*, the outer cover that we know so well.
2. The *dermis*, lying just below the epidermis and known also as the corium.
3. The *subdermis*, a part of the subcutaneous tissue.

The epidermis alone has five distinct layers, or strata (see drawing, page 21), and because we can see only the outside surface it is the one we know and care for—or take for granted and neglect. The dermis, too, gets less gratitude than it deserves. (Its elasticity is a prime factor of a youthful skin.) It contains the sebaceous glands (makers of the body oil, or sebum), the sweat glands, and the hair follicles, which are the shafts in which each hair sits. The vital nerve endings reside there, too. Below the dermis are mainly the fatty tissues, doing important though undramatic work.

The Skin's Basic Duties

The skin is much more than a mere body covering. Its fundamental duties are:

1. *Protection:* it shields us from heat, cold, bacteria, fungi, and other objects in the environment that we are better off without.

2. *Regulation:* it plays a major role in controlling the temperature of the body by maintaining a very uniform inside temperature, regardless of what the temperature is outside.

3. *Respiration:* to some extent the skin "breathes" as the lungs do, taking in oxygen, "exhaling" carbon dioxide, and vaporizing other unwanted gases.

4. *Excretion:* it eliminates sweat, salts, and wastes.

5. *Hydration:* the skin keeps itself soft, smooth, and supple by containing water and by the discharging of perspiration and the oily, sebaceous material that is the skin's best lubricant.

6. *Absorption:* the skin permits certain substances to pass through its tissue, but on a very selective basis. Most harmful substances are kept out, but there are a few exceptions. This capacity of the skin to absorb is being increasingly utilized by physicians for administering medication without injection.

7. *Sensation:* this is achieved by many nerve endings just under the skin's outer surface, making us aware of heat, cold, pressure, and pain, and allowing us to do something about their causes. Sensation acts with lightning speed.

8. *Maintenance of the acid mantle,* a balance between acid and alkali that is preserved on the skin with a trifle more weight on the acid side, to fight off bacterial infection.

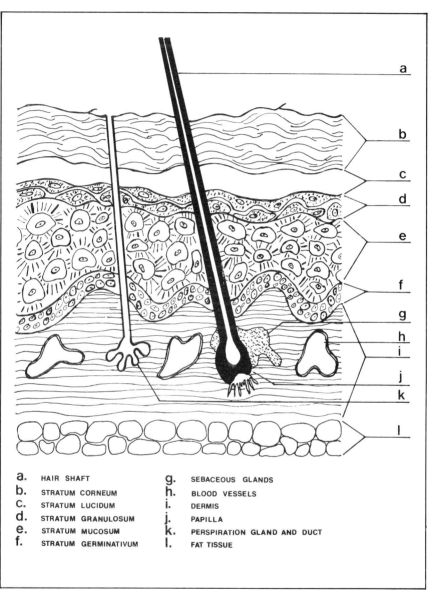

a. HAIR SHAFT	**g.** SEBACEOUS GLANDS
b. STRATUM CORNEUM	**h.** BLOOD VESSELS
c. STRATUM LUCIDUM	**i.** DERMIS
d. STRATUM GRANULOSUM	**j.** PAPILLA
e. STRATUM MUCOSUM	**k.** PERSPIRATION GLAND AND DUCT
f. STRATUM GERMINATIVUM	**l.** FAT TISSUE

Enlarged cross section of the epidermis and dermis.

The Sebaceous Glands

Sebum and its related adjective, *sebaceous,* are key words in this book. They refer to a vital skin function that can be either its boon or its bane. The sebaceous glands in the dermal layer manufacture the body's natural skin oil. These glands are situated just below the surfaces of the face, scalp, ears, neck, and chest, and elsewhere too. This oil, or sebum, constantly replenished, is the lubricant that keeps the skin soft. An over- or undersupply causes the too oily or too dry skin. We'll be mentioning the sebum frequently.

A chemical breakdown shows what sebum is—a complex of fatty acids, both saturated and unsaturated, many organic and inorganic salts, assorted fats, oil, water, miscellaneous debris, and bits of lining discarded by the sebaceous glands.

A red, scaly condition and inflammation around the sebaceous gland openings on the face is known as *seborrhea facialis,* a term that may be translated as excessive excretion of sebum on the face; this is at the root of the inflammation. When the same thing happens on the scalp it is called *seborrhea capitis* (seborrea of the head). This is the basic precondition of dandruff.

Both of these seborrheic conditions, on face or scalp, respond well to an antiseborrheic diet, which is provided elsewhere in this book, and to the external application of an anti-inflammatory liquid or cream, especially one in the corticosteroid family.

When the sebaceous glands are underactive, the skin becomes dry and patchy. This is a condition that benefits from the use of a superfatted soap (nondetergent, containing an increased amount of fats) and an emollient cream. Also helpful during the winter months, when abnormal dryness of the skin is aggravated by overheated and underhumid homes and offices, is a home humidifying device. There are electrical humidifiers on the market, and a basin

of water kept constantly on or under a radiator also works
very nicely.

The Sweat Glands

The sweat glands are of two types, the *eccrine* and
apocrine. The more numerous eccrine glands are tubular
coils based in the middle layer of the skin over almost all
parts of the body. Each gland extends upward through the
skin's top layer, where it forms a pore. The perspiration
excreted through this opening is a clear, thin, watery liquid
that we produce abundantly in warm weather on the forehead, neck, palms, and soles of the feet, and in the armpits.
The sweat from the eccrine glands is about 99 percent
water, and 1 percent inorganic salts and fatty acids. It is
odorless as it emerges from the body, but it picks up an
aroma soon after it is exposed to air. Because an accumula-
tion of it is uncomfortable, we get rid of sweat by air conditioning, fans, or just plain wiping, and ultimately, of
course, by bathing.

A dual function is assigned to the sweat glands. They
carry waste materials from the body, and when perspiration
comes into contact with air, its evaporation has a cooling
effect and acts as a body temperature regulator. In the
course of a winter's day, or on one of low physical activity,
the body will dispose of about a quart (two pounds) of
perspiration. On a day of great heat or great activity, the
output is closer to two quarts.

But it is the apocrine glands that we are more intensely
aware of; they are the reason for the multimillion-dollar
industry that provides the deodorants and antiperspirants.
In short, the apocrine glands are the source of what we call
body odor. They excrete a form of sweat that, while also
originally odorless, is promptly attacked by bacteria
that are always waiting in the warm, moist (and often
hairy) parts of the body; they lose no time in convert-

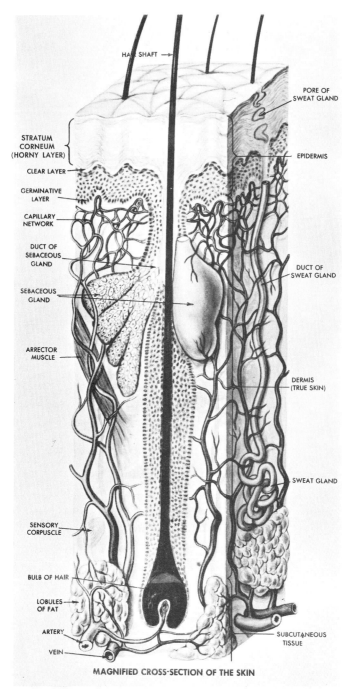

HAIR SHAFT →

PORE OF
SWEAT GLAND

STRATUM
CORNEUM
(HORNY LAYER)

EPIDERMIS

CLEAR LAYER

GERMINATIVE
LAYER

CAPILLARY
NETWORK

DUCT OF
SEBACEOUS
GLAND

DUCT OF
SWEAT GLAND

SEBACEOUS
GLAND

ARRECTOR
MUSCLE

DERMIS
(TRUE SKIN)

SWEAT GLAND

SENSORY
CORPUSCLE

BULB OF HAIR

LOBULES
OF FAT

ARTERY

SUBCUTANEOUS
TISSUE

VEIN

MAGNIFIED CROSS-SECTION OF THE SKIN

(*Courtesy* Today's Health, *American Medical Association*)

Three-dimensional model of a section of
skin, showing its structures.

ing the apocrine sweat into something that is detectably
rancid.

The apocrine glands are situated in a variety of skin
areas but they are most heavily concentrated in the armpits,
the pubic and anal regions, the breasts and navel. They release a viscous liquid—not really a true form of sweat—
that is thicker than the eccrine kind. It is interesting to
note that youngsters who have not yet completed the stage
of puberty, as well as the aged or aging—if they maintain
a reasonably clean state—do not have an odor problem
as a rule. The reason is that at the upper and lower ends
of the age spectrum there is not much perspiring. The ex-
planation of this appears to be related to the sex hormones
—in younger people they are not yet fully active and in
older people their function is waning.

Another intriguing fact is that the sweat caused by heat
or excessive humidity, or both, does not generate nearly as
much odor (nor as quickly) as the sweat produced by
nervousness, fear, or anxiety—on the forehead, neck, palms
of the hands, and even the soles of the feet.

It should also be observed, perhaps on the positive side,
that an apocrine perspiration odor, if it is not too sharp,
may actually be a sort of social advantage. Many people
who detect it in the opposite sex become erotically stimulated by it.

Perspiration plays a distinctly beneficial role as part of a
constant process of the skin. Part of the sweat droplets, as
they emerge, mixes with the oily sebum to form a natural,
beneficial skin lotion.

Deodorants and Antiperspirants: Products sold to combat perspiration odors fall into one of two categories, *anti-*

perspirants and *deodorants.* The essential function of the antiperspirant is to narrow the openings of the sweat pores, which it does with an ingredient called aluminum chlorhydrate. Because bacteria are a basic cause of body odors, antiseptics or antibacterials are added to antiperspirants. An antiperspirant can close the pores for several hours, completely blocking off the perspiration process. In moderate heat, which should produce moderate perspiration, the stoppage may be of no great consequence; but where the suspended sweating would ordinarily be profuse and continuous—or where even moderate sweating is blocked artificially for a few hours—we must face the ultimate fact that *any* forced interference with a natural body process is an open invitation to trouble. In this case, one of the lesser hazards is a heat rash.

The *deodorant* is something else again. For one thing, its ability to handle the entire perspiration problem is more limited than the antiperspirant's. The deodorant's purpose is not to restrict the flow of perspiration but to neutralize the odors it triggers by checking the activity of bacteria and preventing decomposition of sweat. For their antibacterial effect, most deodorants formerly relied heavily upon hexachlorophene, an excellent antibacterial agent, but since the safety of that ingredient has been brought into question, deodorants are more likely to contain TBS (tribromsalicylanilides), or some other phenolic derivatives.

An abnormality that causes excessive sweating can probably be handled effectively by a suitable antiperspirant and/or deodorant. Try a product in one of these two groups, then one in the other, just to determine whether an antiperspirant or a deodorant is more appropriate to your needs. If one type appears superior to the other, experiment further within that product group, trying different brands to find the one that works best for you. (For further information see Chapter 4.)

Perspiration is only one of the skin's excretory responsi-
bilities. In an emergency, the skin will take over the chore
of excretion even from another organ that has become
disabled. Should the vital kidney function, for example,
falter for some reason, the skin will, to the best of its
ability, take up the task of disposing of the body's wastes.
It is not designed to do the whole job of the kidney but to
the extent that it can handle some of that job in a serious
situation, it can make a critical contribution to the pro-
longation of a life.

Your Skin as a Protector

The skin is a loyal servant with an almost endless capacity for enduring with little complaint the outrages to
which we subject it every day—the summer's heat, the
searing sun, the scalding water, the winter's frosts, the
scraping of the daily shave, the tight shoes pinching and
abrading like sandpaper (to say nothing of the barefoot
style's harsh punishments), the household chemicals that
inflame it, the ill-advised use of some cosmetics, the cuts,
the blows, the scrapes, the punctures, and hosts of other
aggressions.

These indignities are inflicted mainly upon the outermost layer, the epidermis, which manages withal to retain
its protective toughness while also remaining soft and
pliant to the touch. The epidermis has a special ability to
adjust itself to the needs and uses of various parts of the
body. Thus it is thinnest on the eyelids, which need instant
flexibility for opening, closing, and blinking, and thickest
on the soles of the feet, which take the full weight of the
body and the endless hammering of walking.

The epidermis, while performing its duty as the body's
outer guard, not only copes with the external assaults but
also flashes warnings that trouble has begun—or is just

beginning—from causes arising either inside or outside the body. The rash, the boil, the inflammation, the bleeding, the small growth—these are not so much disorders or diseases at the visible site as they may be warning symptoms of provocations elsewhere.

However, the day-to-day functions of the skin are performed largely in the invisible layers below the surface, in the dermis and subdermis. Here are housed the tiny mechanisms that create and nourish the hair, and the follicles that give it access to the surface; here, too, are the nerve endings that carry sensation to the brain, which then, accordingly, acts with the speed of light to instruct the muscles on what they must do. Here in this unseen world are the sweat glands that act as a thermal safety valve, the vessels that channel the blood and lymph, the pigment that makes skin light or dark and governs the protective tanning process, the pilomotor muscles that control the movement of the hairs, and the tissues that give the skin the elasticity to preserve, hopefully, a youthful appearance.

These are but some of the aspects of the busy life the skin leads beyond the limits of our sight. We have until now been rather more concerned about what the skin does than about what it is. We can understand both its function and its composition better if we look at a quick inventory of what only one square inch of skin, to its full depth, contains:

19,500,000 cells
65 hairs and muscles
95 to 100 sebaceous (oil) glands
650 sweat glands
19 or 20 blood vessels
78 nerves
78 sensory systems for heat
13 sensory systems for cold
1,300 nerve endings that register pain

19,500 sensory cells at the ends of nerve fibers
160 to 165 pressure complexes for the sense of touch.

The skin, then, can be considered in terms of a complex of small factories, often interrelated, with built-in systems for providing and controlling warmth and cooling, lubrication, fuel supply, waste treatment and disposal, warning alerts, sensing, hair production, intercommunication, and many kinds of automatic controls.

They all are parts of an overall mechanism that is in many respects a living computer, ordering and bringing in materials for stepping up production at one point, diminishing it at another when the need slacks off, and effectively coordinating the entire complex operation.

Sensation and Pain

Probably the least appreciated function of the skin and its systems is the one that enables us to feel pain. Internal organs also are capable of sensing pain, but it is the skin that registers it most often, and for ample reason. The purpose of physical pain, once thought of as divine punishment for some sin, is to preserve or prolong our lives in the face of the many physical adversities that befall us each day.

Pain is what makes you aware that a bee has stung the back of your neck, that you are overexerting yourself dangerously, that an appendix is getting ready to perforate. Pain is nature's warning that something has happened—or is about to happen—that needs looking after at once.

There are rare cases in which an individual is without any capacity for pain. The outlook in such a case is regarded as exceedingly grave.

But pain is only one category of the sensations with which the skin provides us. Sensation is handled by the many nerve endings that lie directly below the skin's surface. They pick up messages that come to the skin from the outside and telegraph them to the brain. The brain, that marvelous computer, translates the messages into language we can understand and flashes them back, usually to muscles, telling us what action should be taken. If we're getting too close to fire—even if we can't see it—the sensation of sudden warmth is a warning. If we get too cold, we have received that message even before the goose bumps (a protective mechanism) appear, and we reach for more covering. Run your finger into a sharp, pointed object and the entire process—nerve message, brain interpretation, and muscle reaction—has jerked your hand away a split second before you even become conscious of what's happened.

Sensation is also an "educator." It teaches us, with time, what dangers must be avoided in order to spare ourselves pain or other disagreeable feelings.

The Intelligent Defender

Of the many defense duties the skin performs for us, the common pressure blister is an outstanding example. Is the blister a nuisance only, or is it a protection?

A man who works at a desk all week goes out of a Saturday to repair some loose pickets in his fence. Not long afterward, a blister rises on his palm or a finger where the hammer handle has exerted greatest pressure. The skin senses that tissues beneath the pressure point have been damaged and it raises a blister, protectively. The blister holds a thin, watery serum intended to cushion the spot against further damage. At the same time, new skin is being formed at the dermal layer and it pushes upward to replace the injured area on the outside. In a few days the new skin presses upward through the watery blister and heals, and the fluid is absorbed. But the skin is wary. Noting that trouble has arisen at this point, the new skin that is formed is somewhat tougher and harder than the old that was damaged.

On the whole, as you must have noticed by now, your skin takes excellent care of you and requires little in return. It will serve you well over a lifetime if you show some occasional concern for it and give it some reasonable minimum of care.

2

"But I Do Have a Good Skin!" Reward It with Care

If you have always had a clear, attractive skin—*almost* always, anyway—be grateful to the parents or parent who conveyed it to you. Be not immoderately proud, for it was not wholly of your own doing.

If you have had to exert some effort to keep it that way, clear and healthful, you may be as proud as you wish. The inheritance is a splendid advantage but it came with no guarantee that you will forever be home-free. To insure this takes some effort.

In an age that has accustomed us to medical marvels, we are inclined to expect a "miracle drug" always to be handy for an instantaneous cure of whatever ails us. That expectation carries over to skin care. The cosmetics market, after all, offers almost daily a new lotion or potion that promises the "ultimate answer" in the quest for skin beauty.

Start with Soap and Water

To keep the skin glowing there is indeed a "miracle drug" better than anything else yet discovered. It has no exotic Latin name. We usually call it soap.

It's strong stuff and requires dilution with a "natural" lotion. That one does have a Latin name, *aqua pura,* but for everyday purposes we call it water.

You don't need a prescription for either of them. All the laboratory equipment needed to blend them is in your bathroom. The only general instruction is that the water be used warm, not hot.

But a warning must be stated here: the use of soap and water may be habit-forming (though some people, especially children, have been known to resist the addiction). In any case, it's the kind of lifetime enslavement that I wholeheartedly endorse.

Of course, not every kind of soap is suitable for everyone, as is made more explicit below, but if none of the exceptions apply to you, forget about them. Wash exposed parts of the body at least morning and night and once in-between if possible. In tub or shower, wash everywhere else, with special attention to armpits, crotch, and chest, giving emphasis to wherever hair grows, however thinly.

Be sure to get all the soap rinsed off well, even though people seen washing or shaving in films generally wipe off the soap with a towel. A few minutes of contact with soap are about all your skin can take, because soap must be mildly alkaline if it is to clean well. Soap is a chemical mixture of fats and alkali. Clear soaps are usually made with a large amount of glycerine replacing much of the fats. This is not the case with detergents.

Note this: unless you have some abnormal perspiration problem, regular use of soap and water will permit you to discard your deodorants and antiperspirants. You'll never miss them.

Just what do soap and water do? To start with, except for special-purpose antiseptic soaps, they do *not* kill germs. But they create an unfavorable environment for them and deprive them of the surroundings in which they thrive and breed.

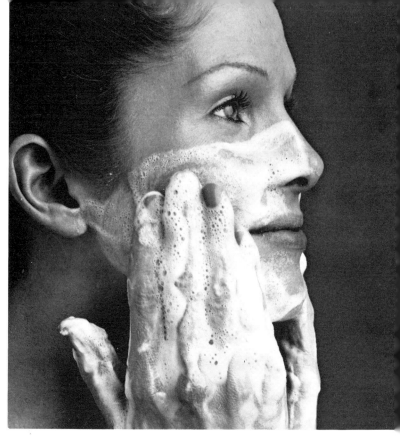

Soap and water are the first and greatest of beauty aids. For washing, a clear soap and warm, not hot water are recommended. If you use a washcloth, do so gently.

Soap's secret weapon is its chains of molecules, which when spread on the skin literally seize and remove everything lying loose on it. The water rinse washes away these loaded soap molecules with everything they carry—dust, grime, grease, city smog, and invisible, used-up cells from the top skin layer, which are always dying and flaking off. Washing with a bit of enthusiasm naturally helps to loosen all that debris. The cargo also includes perspiration and some of the body's natural oil, but these are quickly replaced. The replacement is slower for the aging, who do

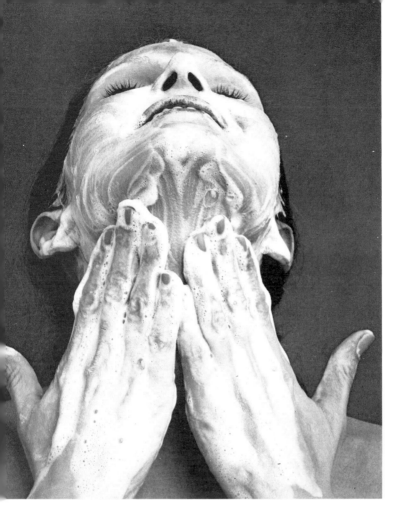

not perspire much, have limited oil production, and should, therefore, limit their bathing. Older people should sometimes use a cleansing cream instead of soap, except for cleaning armpits and crotch.

Choosing a Soap

General precautions in washing include avoiding soaps that are highly alkaline (such as old-style yellow soaps) or heavily perfumed. The first can inflame the skin, the second can oversensitize it to the sun or create other sensitivity problems. Another kind of soap to be used in moderation is the sort containing pumice or other abrasives. Men whose work makes their hands grimy, such as mechanics, may favor the abrasive soaps, but often with injury to the skin. Powdered detergents are made just for such heavy cleansing, and they work well and easily—and safely.

For normal, daily use, the best kind of soap is the simple, white, nonperfumed kind, with some extra assurances offered by a Castile-type soap. The transparent soaps are mild and good cleansers. Ignore the beauty claims of the soap ads. If a soap cleans well and creates no skin problems, expect no more of it than that; it's doing all that soap can do. Its effect on beauty is limited to the fact that no skin can be beautiful unless it is kept clean.

As for the deodorant soaps, they may have an unexpected allergic effect, as explained elsewhere in this volume.

Bathing and Showering

Many widespread ideas about bathing can stand some clarification. From a purely hygienic standpoint, the daily bath is by no means an absolute "must," except, again, in cases of abnormal perspiration. Two or three times a week is quite enough to keep most homemakers or people with office jobs clean and odor-free.

The ritual daily bath is, in fact, largely a bit of modern folklore. It is physically stimulating to some, has an aesthetic value to others, and in either case removes a good deal more sebum, the valuable natural oil, than most of us can spare. I recently heard a television commercial—you may imagine the sponsor's product—that casually assumed that, of course, every responsible woman shampooed every day. That's mischievous nonsense.

It's the kind of subtle arm-twisting advertising that is also pushing the use of bath oils. They are pleasant to use, leaving on the skin a thin film of oil and agreeable fragrance. People with certain severe skin disorders accompanied by serious inflammation are grateful for the temporary relief that bath oils seem to provide. But the benefits of bath oils are only temporary.

The bubble bath is something else. It contains detergent and has been reported to have caused genital inflammation in some children and adults. It confers no benefit whatever on the skin, but it does have a fascination that entices children into a tub. However, a splashing child often gets an eyeful of it and its sting is quite painful. Rubber boats are safer.

It is not necessary to "program" the sequence of events in the process of tub bathing. With the body mostly immersed, do things in the order that comes naturally. However, if a shampoo is one of them, that should be done first, while the water is still clean.

On balance, a shower cleanses better than a tub bath does because the spray helps to loosen up the dirt; besides, sitting in a tub means washing and rinsing with water that is becoming increasingly soiled.

Under a shower, a more exact sequence should be followed in soaping up. Start at the top—with or without shampoo—to avoid having the littered rinse water run down over parts that have already been cleansed. More specifically, that means beginning with washed hands and proceeding downward from face and neck to shoulders, armpits, arms, torso, crotch, thighs, legs, and feet. The shampoo can be a separate operation, performed as desired, but when you are showering all over, and especially when scalp and hair seriously need washing, the shampoo should come first.

The Turkish bath, which uses hot steam, has its devout adherents, but it is more a matter of faith than hygiene. Its extreme heat puts more strain than necessary on the body, especially the heart, and presents even worse hazards when the steaming-hot atmosphere is shifted suddenly to icy-cold. If the only purpose of the Turkish bath or sauna is to get the skin really clean, soap and warm water will do that just as well.

The healthy benefits of the sauna, or Finnish steam bath, have also been greatly overrated. Recently the more limited "facial sauna" has been attracting considerable interest. Its merits, too, have been extravagantly overstated, and little or no mention has been made of a major hazard—the steam may dilate the facial capillaries permanently, leaving a face that is chronically red. Another unpleasant consequence is that the facial sauna accelerates the activity of the sweat glands.

A few generations ago, milk baths were touted as being highly beneficial to the skin (as well as to the renown of stage females who claimed to be addicted to them). More recently, probably due to the "organic" style cycle, the milk bath myth has come around again. If you can afford a tubful of milk and are determined to try it, by all means do. But drink some of it first, because that's the part of the process where the value will be. And afterward, be sure to rinse off very well!

Cleansing Creams and Lotions

After each of your two or three daily washings of the skin with a mild, almost neutral soap, there should be a follow-up with a cleansing cream or liquid, one that is either of the neutral kind or slightly on the acid side to help preserve the skin's protective acid mantle. Cleansing creams can be purchased for normal, dry, and oily skins.

It's pleasant to dus
with bath powder after the bath

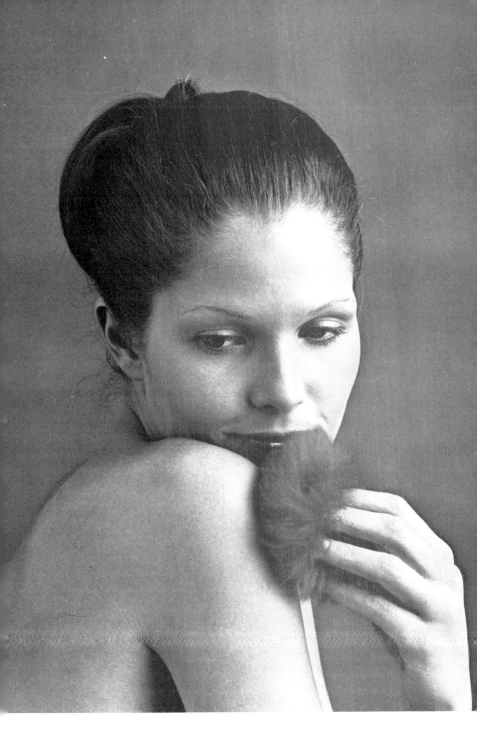

They remove deep-pore dirt, air pollutants, lipstick stains, makeup, and so on, and leave a thin film of emulsified oil on the cutaneous tissues, thus preventing drying of the skin. It is not necessary to purchase expensive cleansing creams, as all of these products are similar in chemical composition and differ only in fragrance and packaging.

Good skin care suggests that if you use foundation makeup, it should be of the non-greasy type. The face powder can be loose or pressed. Makeup should be removed with either a neutral soap, a deep-cleansing cream that contains mineral oil, such as Albolene, or a mild detergent in a cosmetically acceptable cream or emulsion.

After-Cleansing Care

After the makeup has been removed, a stimulating skin freshener may be applied. It is advisable that the kind ordinarily used be nonalcoholic, to avoid excess drying. Occasionally, however, the skin freshener may be replaced by an astringent that does contain some alcohol or witch hazel (also alcoholic) and an antiseptic.

Finally, a mild emollient or moisturizing cream should be lightly dabbed on and stroked gently *away* from the

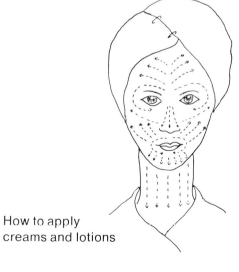

How to apply
creams and lotions

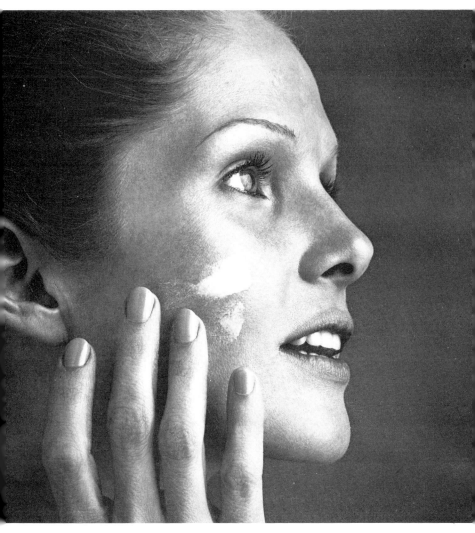

Correctly applying moisturizing cream

center of the face toward the sides. The neck should, of course, be included in the process, and other parts of the body exposed during the day will probably also benefit from the procedure. The eyelids are also important.

Of particular importance is the *frequent* and *faithful* use, in season, of a protective sunscreening cream or lotion containing specific agents that block out the skin-damaging rays of the sun. On any day when exposure to it is significant, the sunscreen should be applied several times. At such a day's end, the skin should be carefully cleansed in the normal way with a lubricating or emollient cream, to reduce the drying effect the sun has exerted, at least to some extent, despite the sunscreening. If the skin is sensitive to the sun, one should use an emollient cream containing a sunscreen such as Reflecta®.

The Dry Skin

A dry skin is one that flakes or chaps often in winter, and sometimes feels tighter than it should. The dryness may be inherited, or it may be caused by a reducing diet that greatly limits or even eliminates fats, which provide nourishment a healthy skin needs. In winter, heat-dried, unhumidified indoor air will also cause a dry skin. If you have a dry skin, follow the directions given in Chapter 13, "Your Skin in Winter."

Cleansing Review

In sum, then, there are a few basic aids that you should use regularly and properly for a smooth and supple skin. You will probably be using others, too, but they will be more for decorative purposes than for skin care. For ideal care, the essentials are:

1. Soap and water
2. Cleansing cream or liquid cleanser
3. Makeup remover
4. Skin freshener (nonalcoholic)
5. Moisturizing cream.

Gloves That Help Red Hands

A different type of product has proved helpful in reducing a frequent source of embarassment—redness and roughness of the hands. This is Spandex gloves, worn at night. I evaluated the wearing of these gloves in a recent study and found that in a majority of the patients the redness and roughness of the hands were diminished. This result was considered to be due to the isotoner effect—the continuous, gentle pressure of the synthetic elastic fibers exerting a protective and massaging effect. The softening effect is enhanced by applying under the gloves a penetrating cream containing a polymer that acts as a protective agent. A beneficial side effect was the improvement of arthritic and rheumatoid twinges of pain—probably due to the invisible, continuous, massaging effect of this miracle material. Incidentally, the gloves are made in all colors, so that they can be also used during the day, to match one's costume. A complete body suit is now being sold for a similar stimulating effect upon the skin of the entire body.

A Note on Skin Cleansing for Men

The previous advice pertains mostly to women. This book is written for men too, more information for them on skin care will be found in Chapter 5, which deals with skin and hair aids for men. Suffice it to say here that regular washing with a mild soap is necessary two to three times a day. A thin, absorbable moisturizer should be applied at night and after sunning. This will have the additional benefit of softening the beard, reducing the havoc of its bristles upon the skin of the female partner during those romantic moments.

There's More to It than Cleansing

Soap, water, and other cleansing aids are not, of course, the whole story of maintaining an attractive skin, but when we get beyond that point the options become confusing; the breadth of choices, stridently proposed, is overwhelming. The exploitation of hope rolls on without restraint. In her book *World of Beauty,* Edith Serei writes: "Those who offer 'miracle' beauty treatments that restore youth and beauty in a matter of hours or days prove by their very claims that they are charlatans of the worst kind." I heartily agree with this viewpoint.

Achieving a healthful and attractive skin demands effective daily care, with special emphasis on cleansing, as I have already stressed, but it also requires a balanced and nourishing diet with vitamins and trace mineral supplements, adequate body exercise, balanced emotional attitudes, and a hopeful mental outlook. Facial isometric exercises and mild massage are also helpful.

These requisites are not necessarily stated in the order of their importance, for it is not possible to assign such priorities. *All* of them are necessary for making the most of one's features, and the omission of one of them can make the other practices futile.

We'll take up cosmetic aids fully in Chapters 4 and 5, and the vital subject of diet in Chapter 7.

3

Acne: Skin Disorder
of the Teen-Ager

The proper control of skin disorders among teen-agers is a matter of special urgency. Acne and other chronic skin ailments, even when especially associated with youth, can be carried into advanced adulthood, or if not the disease itself, then the scarring and pitting that often result. These unsightly consequences become more serious as our society places increasing stress on beauty and youthful appearance. These may be overemphasized, but that is no consolation to a young woman with otherwise attractive features whose facial scars, no matter how slight, may produce a far graver pattern of permanent psychological scarring.

Except for the hippy minority, young people today subscribe to a culture in which personal appearance—clothing, skin, hair—plays a highly prominent role. The achievement of personal attractiveness requires a special commitment to good habits, and this in turn demands a measure of self-discipline. From both standpoints, the goal is eminently worth seeking.

It is generally accepted that teen-agers, though many of them would be the last to agree, have a special need for mature understanding, guidance, practical cooperation and, where indicated, a bit of prudent nudging. The teen years are most highly regarded by older adults as a carefree

45

time marked by a lack of grown-up responsibility; but they forget the aching confusions of being neither an adult nor a child, of the surging new sex drives and other sudden physical phenomena that the youngster hasn't learned to direct or control. Adolescence can be a period of great emotional turbulence. The turmoil is usually concealed (more or less) until time establishes (more or less) a more mature balance. What elude concealment are the sorry by-products of the inner turmoil: the skin disorders— the acne, the too-dry skin, the too-oily skin, the excessive dandruff (seborrhea). They are worn openly on face and scalp, and a swimsuit may reveal them even more glaringly.

What Causes Acne?

Acne is by far the most prevalent of these disorders. By some estimates, as many as 90 percent of teen-agers endure it to some extent. It is essentially a disorder of the sebaceous glands, lying just below the top layer of the skin, which manufacture and distribute sebum. In adolescence these glands often become overactive. Sometimes, though more rarely, this happens in later life. It is triggered by the vigorous hormonal changes that are taking place and stimulated further by a combination of emotional factors and the deplorable standard teen diet, which centers on excessive starches, fats, spices, iodized salt, sweets, and shellfish.

Consider the beloved hamburger, which usually has a 25 to 35 percent fat content and is often fried in more fat; the spicy hot dog, for which the law has only recently set an appalling 30 percent maximum of fats, and the mustard or spicy relish that goes with it; the high-butterfat milk shake; the pizza with its starch, cheese, spices and probably iodized salt; and the "shrimp basket," another acneprovoker like all shellfish, except that this one is fried in deep fat, salted and drenched in highly spiced sauce. Don't exclude eggs, usually scrambled, served with starchy fried potatoes and garnished with ketchup.

Some physicians believe acne is unrelated to diet; others hold that it is aggravated by all these fatty, starchy, and spicy foods. Experience has committed me to the latter view.

The Cycle of Acne

The behavioral causes of acne are quite well known; the basic underlying cause—what it is that the apparent causes have in common—is not. But the life cycle of acne is otherwise no mystery.

Regarding young people, some generalizing is permissible. Their hormonal glands, which have just become fully operative, tend to overdo matters; they become excessively active. They overstimulate the release of sebum, making the skin too greasy (they can come up with a total fresh supply every three hours). The hormonal glands produce enough sebum to plug up the sebaceous gland openings on the skin. When a plugged duct stops flowing it touches off an unhappy sequence of events. First, a whitehead (*milia*) becomes visible just under the skin surface. As it emerges and becomes exposed to air it quickly oxidizes and becomes a blackhead (*comedone*). It often happens that the skin's hardened (horny) top layer has grown over the duct outlet and further blocked it, and if there is no quick release of the blockage the result is a red, raised bump, commonly called a pimple (*comedone*). By any name, it's an infection, and the body's defense system rushes white blood cells to the afflicted area. As they join battle with the invading bacteria, pus forms; the result is now the unlovely and infectious skin lesion known as a pustule or a pus pimple.

In time, the evidence of a bout of acne may vanish, but it may also leave a face pitted or pockmarked, or both. The outcome depends on how the infection has been handled. A family physician or dermatologist is almost sure to cope with it successfully except in a few obstinate cases, and even these can be controlled.

Home treatment, as we shall see, can also be effective when the disorder is a moderate one. The problem here is that the treatment chosen usually consists of squeezing the pimple to release the infectious matter. That technique can be disastrous, because it will usually spread the infection.

Prevention and Control of Acne

The best answer lies in prevention, and that demands persistence, patience, and discipline. Here are some broad guidelines:

Keep washing an oily skin as many times a day as it takes to maintain an oil-free condition. Wash all oily areas—forehead, face, neck, back, shoulders, chest, and upper arms. Do it gently—repeat, *gently*. A detergent soap, because of its drying effect, is better than ordinary soap with its fatty base. What makes oily skin a serious matter is that it offers the richest soil for the cultivation of acne bacteria.

What the oily skin does not need is more grease. So be very sparing with cold cream or creamy cosmetics. Better yet, don't use them at all.

Do not pick at or squeeze a pimple. Even freshly washed fingers are not sterile enough to guard against further infection at the site or by spreading to adjacent tissue. The only acceptable home treatment is to soak sterile pads in hot water and apply them to the affected area (avoiding finger contact). Though many physicians distrust advertised remedies, I believe that in *very mild* cases of acne, any of the chemist's antiacne preparations may be tried for brief periods. They usually contain drying agents that can be helpful but will surely bring no permanent cure. Only medical care can do that.

Shampoo the scalp regularly because it, too, has sebaceous glands producing oil. Where there is acne there is also likely to be oily hair, and its burden of grease and grime, inevitably touching the skin below the hair line, contributes to the acneous condition. Use a detergent shampoo or one made for oily scalps—but *never* an oily shampoo.

Special Note: Long hair styles can be the best friend acne ever had. The long hair always touches the forehead, parts of the face, and even the shoulders. Thus, long hair must be kept flawlessly clean—by frequent shampooing.

Watch that diet. Forget that nuts, iodized salt, and chocolates ever existed. Avoid all other fats and oils, including fatty meats and dairy products. Spices are no friends either. Watch for a possible relationship between an acne flare-up and a specific food you've eaten; the flare-up might be an allergic reaction to it.

Live as your good sense dictates. Get regular exercise, especially outdoors, plenty of rest and sleep, and regulate your diet to avoid constipation. About constipation: as we have seen, the skin excretes, too, and when constipation locks in the body's wastes they tend to seek the skin as an outlet for release. Where acne is already present, the result can be pretty untidy. "Strong" laxatives may seem to help on a one-shot basis, but if used often they actually upset the system and invite more constipation. The answer here, too, lies in exercise, fresh vegetables and fruits, and drinking enough water. Prunes, prune juice, yogurt, and bulky cereals also are effective.

Analyze your anxieties. Aren't they mostly worries that time will take care of? They usually are. As I've noted, acne usually comes with the activation of the sex hormone glands, and one result is a prevailing sense of emotional disquiet, which tends to worsen the acne in a kind of vicious cycle. And so, sorting out the anxieties and evaluating them realistically is guaranteed to be beneficial.

While general rules for the prevention or control of acne are the same for boys and girls, in some respects the causes and effects of acne are different in the two sexes. Boys are more likely to get it—and get it more severely. Yet boys also worry less about it than girls do, understandably. Boys are more susceptible because acne is associated with special activity of the male hormone (testosterone). On the other hand, the dominant female hormone (estrogen) clearly tends to control acne. Girls should understand this clearly because it will avoid worry if the skin erupts a bit a few days before the menstrual cycle begins. At that time the estrogen production is at its lowest point in the twenty-eight-day cycle, which means a weakening of this natural defense against acne. The skin will probably clear up in a few days with little help.

In stubborn cases of acne in girls, a new and effective control has been discovered. Dr. John S. Strauss of the Boston University Medical Center has reported that even a very small quantity of a highly active estrogen product called *ethynyl estradiol* brings a significant decrease in sebum production, to the benefit of acneous or very oily skin.

Interestingly, the Strauss team has resorted to the chemical formula of the contraceptive pill and its pattern of use to combat acne. Either the estrogen—the Pill's major ingredient—is combined in a pill with progestin, or the two hormones are taken in separate pills in a certain sequence during the menstrual cycle. However, the estrogen is apparently the ingredient of prime value.

Word has gotten around among young people that the contraceptive pill is a sure-fire cure for acne. The Pill is not aspirin. Its indiscriminate, unsupervised use can cause tragedies far worse than acne. It cannot be used without the prescription of a doctor who will check the patient regularly for evidence of serious reactions.

Under no conditions should boys use the Pill—and there are reports that some do—unless they don't care about its feminizing effects. It can impair their masculinity, perhaps permanently. Nor may girls under sixteen take it lest normal bone growth be arrested. It must be noted that Dr. Strauss does not use estrogen for acne unless all the more conventional treatments have failed; even with the estrogen it generally takes a few months before results are observed. The treatment, he reports, can help to suppress new outbreaks but does not improve lesions already existing.

However, other approaches to acne control, even in stubborn cases, have been used effectively by family physicians and dermatologists.

Another avenue of fresh hope has been opened up by Dr. Ruth K. Freinkel, a Harvard dermatologist, whose experiments have suggested a relationship between acne pimples, pustules and cysts, and concentrations of free fatty acids in the skin. When she injected such acids into the skin, acne erupted at the site.

Dr. Freinkel and associates from the Harvard and Boston University medical schools found that some antibiotics, notably tetracycline, reduced the acid concentrations. The weakening caused the oily sebum to lose a great deal of its ability to trigger an acne eruption. There was an additional plus: the type of bacterium dominant in acne, known as *cornybacterium acnes,* is quickly laid low by such antibiotics as tetracycline.

Thus numerous techniques and medications are available to the doctor in treating acne. He may elect to open a pustule surgically and drain it, which is simple and painless and best left to him. A dermatologist may use superficial x-ray treatments that shrink the size and activity of the sebaceous glands, or he may prescribe the use of Vitamin A. Another approach is with ultraviolet light, which tends to peel off the outer layer of skin, thereby helping clear an unsightly patch as well as opening up plugged glands so that they drain off their infected contents. Acne usually shows great improvement in the summer when the skin is exposed to the sun's natural ultraviolet rays, which are superior to those of the ultraviolet lamp. But exposure to the sun should not be excessive.

In addition to any or all such forms of treatment, the dermatologist will prescribe one of a number of chemical formulas for direct application to the eruptions. It will peel the skin or shrink the pustules, or both. This is likely to be a lotion containing precipitated sulfur, salicylic acid, and resorcin. Also prescribed will probably be a soapless detergent, medicated cleansers, and drying agents. Treatment will vary among patients according to many individual factors that only a doctor can detect and manage.

Occasionally a severe or long-lasting acne infection will leave distressing residual scars. They need not be endured, for they can be removed by dermabrasion (skin-planing) or chemosurgery (peeling). These treatments demand skill of a high order and should be performed only by a dermatologist trained in these techniques (as most are). Even the most expert treatment is not without some discomfort, but those who have experienced it think the results are worth it. Sometimes a procedure must be repeated for the best effect.

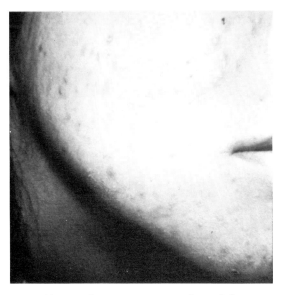

Above: A severe case of pustular acne. *Below:* The same young man's face after eight weeks' treatment.   (AUTHOR'S COLLECTION)

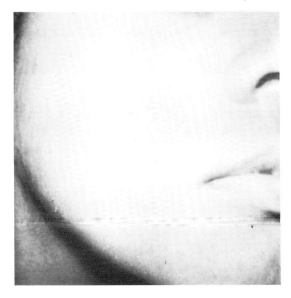

Oily Skin Without Acne

An oily skin, to which young adults are prone, may be free of acne only because the oil is fortunately lacking in the yet-unknown chemical or pathological factor that is the essence of acne. No one should assume that immunity to acne is permanent; the oily skin is often its forerunner. Oily skin should therefore be approached with all of the measures already outlined for the preventive control of acne—scrupulous hygiene, adequate rest and sleep, regular exercise, avoidance of anxieties to whatever extent is possible, and in general, prudent and moderate living habits.

All fried and other fatty foods must be shunned.

The oily skin is easily noticed because even the dimmest light will reflect the shiny sebum on the forehead, nose, cheeks, or chin. The constant flow of oil is likely to be controlled by frequent washing with a medicated or soapless detergent cleanser or a soap which emulsifies the fat. These should be used as often as six times a day, if needed, and always generously rinsed away. After rinsing, freshen your skin with a mild astringent containing witch hazel, diluted alcohol, and perhaps a degreasing chemical like acetone, or dilute alcohol and an allantoin derivative. Women may then apply a makeup foundation for oily skin. If during the morning or afternoon oil is present in large quantities, dab the area with a tissue or a liquid towelette containing acetone. Acetone will readily remove the oil. Then reapply astringent, following with a nonoily foundation or face powder. Several types of "wipe and dry" towelettes are available.

At night, I suggest the use of an abrasive that contains a cleansing agent, an abrasive such as aluminum oxide, polyethylene (plastic) particles, or pumice and antiseptic.

The face is moistened, the cleansing abrasive is used to remove grime, oil, and debris, and it is left on the face for
two minutes, then washed off. A therapeutic drying agent
is then used. Some popular products are Pernox®,
Brasivol®, Dermabrade®, Ionax®.

If back or shoulders show excessive oil, use the same
cleansing procedures, but with a long-handled brush of
natural bristles or with a *natural* sponge.

Sometimes oily skin may occur with an oily scalp because some similar factor is at work in both cases. For the
oily skin I also counsel frequent shampooing, on the order
of every three days. The shampoo must be made especially
for oily hair or scalp and should contain a small measure
of alcohol and *triethanolamine,* an alkali that handles oil
well by emulsifying it.

A frustrating form of excessive oiliness is the patchy
combination type—too oily here, too dry in adjacent spots.
The oily area may go down the center of the face, across
forehead, nose and chin, with the rest of the face either
normal or even dry. The oily spots should be treated carefully and locally. The entire face is first washed with a mild
cleanser; then the oil spots alone are washed with pads
soaked in alcohol and an antiseptic. As for a foundation, a
single lotion is not likely to be suitable for both dry and
oily skin, so it seems best to use an absorbent pressed
powder on the oily places and cover the rest of the face
with a light-textured, matte foundation, either liquid or
cream.

Some Minor Comfort for the Acne-Afflicted

Do your date and acne eruption arrive at the same time? Foundation makeup of your own flesh tone will carry you through the evening without risk.

If all else fails, implore the intervention of St. Procopius. Although I have made futile efforts to confirm it, he is said to be the patron saint of acne. If this early Christian martyr had acne, it vanished when he lost his head in A.D. 303.

4

Beauty and Cosmetics

Since the poet John Davies advanced the notion about 1616, beauty has often been considered in terms of a single, tissue-thin dimension—"skin deep." The dermatologist, however, can assure you that authentic beauty is not at all skin deep—the truest kind of beauty is not achieved by applying something externally, but consists in an indefinable quality of personality or spirit originating inside, rising mysteriously to the surface, and enduring for a lifetime.

A woman's beauty is related to her personality, her figure, carriage, speech, and wardrobe, as well as to the appearance of her skin. With good taste and experience, however, any woman can enhance the beauty of her skin through the proper use of cosmetics.

Columnist Harriet Van Horne has pointed out that many of the high-priced cosmetics may not smoothe away the wrinkles or convert the blemished skin into a baby's, but while the purchaser may know that very well, what she is buying is hope. Since all of us lead lives that are less than perfect and seldom see our most cherished goals realized, buying hope at that price seems a good bargain. Like truth, hope dashed to earth rises again. Involved with cosmetics are some undashable truths, too. Remember them:

• Cosmetics *can* help make you more attractive, though they are, at best, only "beauty aids."

• Treat them like strong medicine—if a little helps, doubling the dose will defeat your purpose.

From France and Switzerland come many cosmetic products containing exotic but scientifically unproved compounds. Among them are royal jelly, pollen, placenta extract, and other so-called biological stimulants. Extracts from animal cells are used both internally and externally. Their efficacy is similarly unproved.

The daily practice of skin hygiene adds to the value of cosmetics. All you will need to know about the usefulness of cosmetics is contained in this chapter. That is not an exaggerated claim, because there is really not too much, beyond the basic facts listed here, that you will find helpful. Anything else is likely to be unrelated to your situation and needs, unless they are most unusual.

That may seem a gross oversimpification of a complex subject if you are a reader of the vast volume of "beauty" journalism produced every day of the year by newspaper and magazine assembly lines. Much of it is sound and commendable, written by responsible people who avoid recommendations, implied or explicit, of scientifically unproved products and practices. Others warn sternly against such life-or-death acts as cutting your hair except on astrologically sanctioned days—or at specified hours, which in one instance fell between midnight and dawn.

Others write rhapsodically of unrestricted sunbathing and its unmatched health benefits, even though it is now quite firmly established that excessive sun exposure (and "excessive" isn't very much) is *the* leading cause of premature and irreversible skin aging, solar keratoses (precancerous), and probably of skin cancer and a disturbing list of other stubborn, unsightly skin disorders.

Today most cosmetics are manufactured under sterile conditions, using pure chemicals. They are tested by trained dermatologists and can be used safely to make the skin more attractive. Similar products from different manufacturers do sometimes vary in price. This is usually due to higher expenditures by one of the companies for packaging, advertising, research, or scientific staff.

We find in the press laudatory accounts of the new "natural" cosmetics that contain extracts from fruits and vegetables, spices, and oils pressed from plants. At best, these "natural" and "organic" ingredients are probably harmless—except to skins sensitive to one or more of them. Their value in softening the skin, removing wrinkles, or imparting the glow of health has not been proved. The ads and press stories about them do not warn of the allergic reactions they may trigger.

Cosmetic dermatitis is discussed in Chapter 6.

The search for beauty is now extended into more advanced years than it once was, and properly so. It is also beginning earlier. As this was being written, a quite respectable cosmetics company announced it was bringing out a line of cosmetics for sophisticated women—in the eight-to-sixteen-year bracket. At least two established concerns now produce an impressive range of cosmetics for men. My concern in this chapter will be primarily with women's cosmetics. I'll discuss those for men in the next chapter.

The word "cosmetic" is derived from a Greek word meaning simply "adornment." A few centuries ago, powder and rouge were the only available adornments for the skin. Today there has been a vast increase in the number of types of cosmetic products available.

The term "cosmetic" is also used as an adjective, in a figurative sense. Thus to dress up a company's account books to conceal bad news is called "cosmetic book-keeping."

The kind of cosmetics bought today, of course, range far beyond mere powder and rouge, and the scope of the term is pretty flexible. A hair-coloring rinse, which helps to adorn, is of course a cosmetic; but so is a perfume, which appeals only to the sense of smell and not to the eye. Even a foundation cream, neither seen nor smelled, is accepted as a cosmetic.

Once, "cosmetic skin" was an unsightly ailment caused by overuse of chemically harsh rouge or perhaps by an allergic reaction to a cosmetic, but little was then known about that. Though cosmetic skin is little seen today—because cosmetics are now of far higher quality and women have learned to handle them better—allergies still occasionally occur. Quality is better because the manufacturers, with much at stake, allot large sums to chemical research. Indeed, they cannot afford to do less. Their drive to broaden their product ranges, however, has resulted in wide duplication of quite similar products, each touted as being unique, and they bear individual brand names giving no clue to the fact that they actually may be simple, familiar formulas, perhaps slightly modified. Most of them have another common quality: they are highly over-priced.

This desire to sell goods has not been without public benefits. For one thing, some of the products when properly used do indeed help to beautify, bringing to the user an additional psychological boon that cannot be shrugged off. Equally important, cosmetic advertising, though not informative, has made women beauty-conscious and thereby hygiene-conscious as well.

What Cosmetics Do

We know that wholesome cosmetics, properly used, protect the skin from excessively cold and from impure or dry air, thus keeping it younger longer. But in the past decade or so another use has appeared, along with a new skin hazard. In that period our population balance has shifted from rural to urban, while cities have been producing an increasing number and range of air pollutants that severely attack skin health. This new condition, for which I have chosen the descriptive term "City Skin," is marked by redness, surface irregularities, and chronic inflammation. Special cosmetics are useful in controlling and preventing it or in causing it to abate. These subjects are discussed in Chapter 12. I have also described this condition in its scientific aspects in the medical journal *Clinical Medicine*.

For this and other day-to-day skin needs there are innumerable cosmetic preparations, well known under many brand names, that will:

- Cleanse the skin
- Lubricate a dry skin or degrease one excessively oily
- Prepare it properly for final makeup
- Protect it from sun damage.

Cosmetics and Skin Tolerance

Allergic reactions to cosmetics can be baffling, but a simple understanding of how—though not exactly why—they happen is possible.

"But how can I be allergic to that cold cream?" a patient protested. "I've been using that brand for six years and it's been just fine. The eruptions must be due to something else."

Those six "safe" years had not, as she thought, proved her immunity; on the contrary, they had slowly built up a sensitivity to that brand of cream. Sometimes, of course, a manufacturer changes a formula, adding something new against which some people's skin rebels.

It's because such sensitivity can build up over a long period that a cosmetic product may, after a long delay, start bringing numerous complaints of allergic reactions even though the maker has diligently pretested it on one hundred or two hundred volunteers with no adverse effect whatever. But his test subjects could give only a week or two to the trials; had the tests lasted six to twelve months, some of the subjects would probably have developed a visible intolerance to the product.

An especially troublesome allergic reaction, because it is often difficult to run down, is frequently caused by nail polish. When it appears clearly in the fingertip area, the cause is obvious. But it is just as likely to show up in more remote parts of the body.

One woman came to my consulting room with a persistent rash on and near her eyelids. It seemed no ordinary dermatitis, so she was advised to abandon her eyelash makeup, the logical villain. That didn't help matters. The rash spread to her chin—but the *right* side only—and in a few weeks it was on her chest, under the left armpit, and then in the ano-genital area. During her first visit I had begun a series of standard patch tests to narrow down the suspected causes. All proved negative and it was certainly not possible to point a finger at any of her facial cosmetics. I knew I had to pick up another trail. One day as we sat talking across my desk, I noticed something. The patient, a some-

what tense and nervous lady, raised her right hand frequently to scratch her right eyelid, then the right side of
her face. And then the left armpit. It seemed a wholly in-
voluntary and unconscious act. I asked whether scratching
was a regular habit.

"Only when I'm feeling anxious," she said. "At home,
when I have some clothes off, I scratch other places, too—
not hard, though."

True, the rashes did not appear to be scratch-induced.
Then I had it. I suggested she bring in her nail polish and
tested it on her shoulder. A rash appeared in forty-eight
hours. I mentioned a few brands of hypoallergenic nail
polish, which protect against reactions, and while I am
quite sure I did nothing to end her scratching, it became
immediately possible for her to enjoy her habit, one might
say, without blemish.

We shall discuss cosmetic dermatitis and allergies in
more detail in Chapters 6 and 11.

Cosmetics: Their Infinite Variety

Among our abundant riches, few match the profusion of
goodies offered by the cosmetic shelves. So rapidly do new
ones appear that a woman who resolved to try them all
would discover, after a lifetime of effort, that the number
still untried kept increasing.

You really need to buy only a few of them—perhaps a
half-dozen. The rest are a waste of time and money, unlikely
to add anything of value to your few basics. Stay with the
brands you like, preferably as low-cost as you can find.
(Manufacturers often turn out the same product under
different labels—one for the expensive boutique, the other
for the cheaper stores.) Change if you develop an un-

pleasant allergic reaction (more about this in Chapter 11), for here it's far better to switch than fight.

While it is by no means recommended that you use them all, let us lift the confusing veil of glamour from some of the most common types of cosmetics and identify them for what they really are:

Soap, while often sold as a beautifier or deodorizer, has only one real function—to clean. True, there are different types for dry or oily skin or hair. If a soap produces an allergy, it is usually due to the alkali or perfume in it. Soap is a broad term that often includes detergents, which are actually soapless. Many products sold as soap actually contain synthetic cleaners. They are often used by industrial workers to remove grime and stains from their hands.

Face powders contain several powdered chemicals, notably talcum, plus a rougelike coloring agent. With the cake form, which is a compressed powder, a moist puff is used. Men's after-shave powder is usually a scented talcum.

Foundation lotion is a specially formulated, liquified face powder suspended in alcohol, glycerin and, perhaps, water. It comes in a range of colors and is quick-drying. The lotion—or the heavier foundation cream—is used as a foundation for powder or other makeup because it leaves a dull finish, giving them better adherence. It also provides a good "cover" for blemishes. A *foundation stick* consists of hard, concentrated lotion ingredients and is used for pinpoint coverage of small blemishes.

Rouge is one of the oldest cosmetics. It consists of a powder base to which a natural tint has been added. It is still among the most useful aids for bringing a temporary touch of color to the skin. It should be used sparingly and is best applied with a brush made for the purpose. Rouge comes in cakes, liquid, and powder form. There are count-

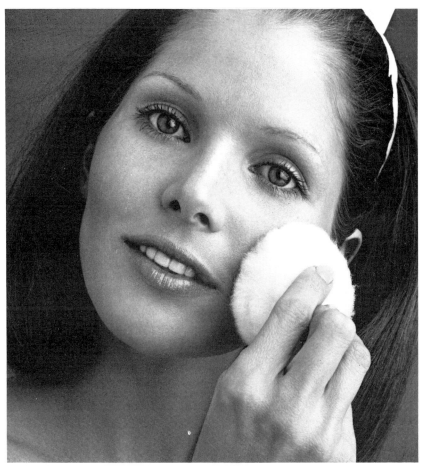

How to apply a powder foundation to the face

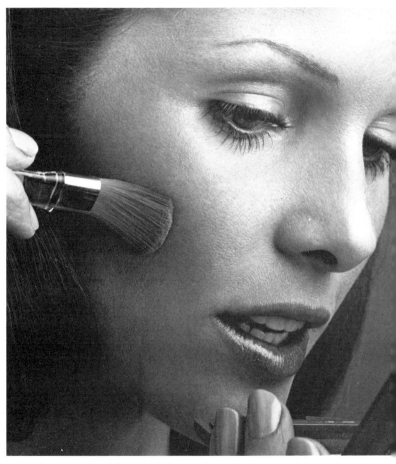

Rouge should be applied with a brush made for the purpose.

less shades to match any complexion. Rouges are also called "blushers."

Lipsticks, the world's richest source of color names, are a blend of beeswax, lanolin, dye, and hectic sales promotion. The so-called permanent lipsticks provide a coating that stays fresh longer than others but may have a drying effect. Some lipsticks use more oil to produce a shine, but these need to be renewed more often. "Liquid lip cosmetic," applied with a brush, is becoming more popular. The dye in any lip rouge may occasionally bring on allergic rash. In that case, change both brand and type at once.

Eye shadow comes in either cream or a dry form. Containing a dye, it is used over the upper eyelid. Shades are numerous. Darkening the upper part of the eyelid makes natural dark circles underneath them less noticeable. Used with restraint, eye shadows can lend a certain allure.

Eyeliner, also a dye, is available with either a cream or

Correct use of an eyeliner

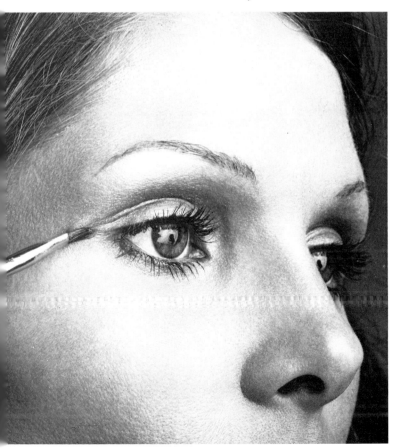

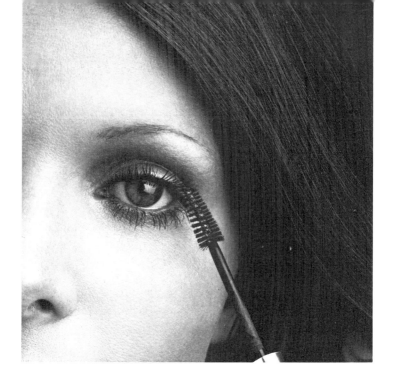

Above: Mascara lends the eyelashes a longer, lusher effect. *Below:* Allure can also be quickly added to the eye by applying artificial eyelashes.

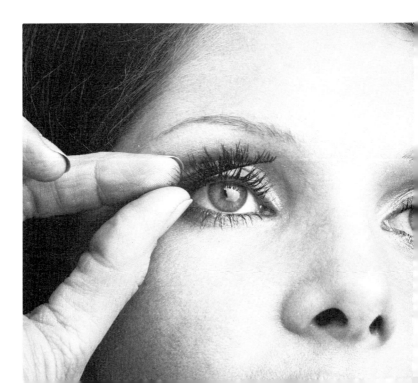

liquid base and there is a pencil form, too. As with eye shadows, eyeliners come in many shades. Liner is applied on the edge of the upper lid, creating an illusion of thicker lashes. Used artfully, it changes the apparent shape of the eye and adds allure.

Eyebrow pencils are very soft pencils with heavy dye ingredients that give the eyebrows a lusher, more emphatic appearance.

*Eyelash makeup—mascara—*is a dye-bearing cream that beautifies pale or sparse lashes. Present formulas are regarded as wholly safe. Mascara is applied with special brushes.

Astringents close open "pores" and tighten the skin temporarily. Ordinary, inexpensive witch hazel is about as good an astringent as any; scented alcohol will do nicely too. Most astringents sold in more elegant packaging contain scented alcohol. If you prefer, you can scent your own witch hazel or rubbing alcohol with perfume, though the branded varieties often include another antiseptic too. If a razor nick is not too deep, an astringent will stop the bleeding. It is a good cleaner for oily skin and an excellent skin freshener.

Emollient cream usually contains lanolin and petrolatum, though quite often other fats, oils, and waxes are used instead. It has a most benign softening effect on the skin and is indispensable in any cosmetics kit. Emollient cream is good for dry skin. It is sold also under such descriptions as night cream, softening cream, lubricating cream—even eye cream and throat cream.

Moisturizing cream acts as a conditioner for tired, dry, parched skin. It helps retain the skin's moisture and thus its elasticity—the most vital quality of a young skin. Emulsion moisturizers are oil and water mixtures and are usually used under makeup. "Humectant" moisturizers are greaseless but leave a thin protective film on the skin's surface to keep moisture in. They may be used either alone or under makeup.

Hand creams and hand lotions are preparations that curb chapping, dryness, and skin irritations. They are made of oil (vegetable or mineral), lanolin, cholestrin, alcohol, water, and emulsifying agents that bind them all together. Recent helpful additions are Vitamins A, D, and E, urea, and often other chemicals—individually or in combinations.

Cold cream, an old, all-purpose stand-by, is as effective as ever for temporary softening of skin and removing makeup. Its usual formula includes beeswax, borax, oil, water, and alcohol. With only slight changes in the formula it becomes an emollient cream.

Cleansing lotion consists mainly of a detergent with an oil that boosts its cleansing effectiveness. It will do a fast job of makeup removal, but soap and water will do it just as well, though perhaps not with the same speed. Similar preparations are available in cream form.

Nail polish consists of resins, synthetic rubber, and a hardening agent. Nail-hardening polishes can be useful in protecting "soft" nails or those prone to splitting, but they sometimes set up a cosmetic dermatitis. Users should watch nails and fingernail area closely for any reaction.

"Natural" Cosmetics: Pay Your Money and Take Your Choice

No doubt it has been the sudden, explosive interest in environmental purity that has turned so many otherwise sober citizens into dedicated seekers of all things "natural," first in foods and more recently in cosmetics. What is undeniably natural is that there should be their exploiters waiting for these folks. Quite ordinary foods, grown in the usual ways, are often sold as "organic" foods at prices

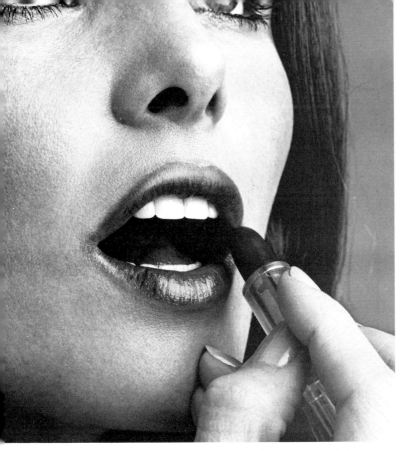

Correct covering of lips with lipstick

double or triple what they would otherwise bring. The most that can be said for them is that they may give the purchaser the illusion of improved health.

In my experience, the "natural" cosmetics have been even more questionable. Consider the types advertised—strawberry, cucumber, honey, skim milk, apple, assorted fruits, and herb. Extracts of the fruit, vegetable, or herb are used in preparing natural cosmetics. If the "flavors" just mentioned—which seem more appropriate for jelly than for a face cream—were in fact "natural" rather than synthetic, that in itself might be dangerous. A woman who eats some cucumber every few weeks may tolerate it very well, but keeping it on her skin for hours, perhaps every day, would be quite another matter. The skin might easily become sensitized to it in a few weeks.

There are other objections to these "natural" cosmetics that go even deeper. First, none of them is truly "natural," nor can it be. Even if one of its ingredients is indeed a freshly picked cucumber, as advertised, a usable product takes more than that—it needs chemical agents to bind the other ingredients together, to emulsify and suspend them. They are pretty sure to include lanolin and emulsifying agents. Without such commonly used chemicals the cosmetic wouldn't work. The secret of making a better cosmetic generally lies in the art of manufacture rather than in the ingredients. A well-established cosmetic concern employs specialized chemists who belong to the Society of Cosmetic Chemists of the United States. The author is a member of this organization.

There is an even more basic question: What is a cosmetic's function? It is expected only to adorn superficially —to make some bodily feature *look* a bit better, and then only temporarily. It does not actually *alter* that feature in the least, nor should it. To do that the cosmetic would have to penetrate far beneath the skin's outer layer and then work some wondrous magic. Any product that tried to do that would be extremely hazardous. None of them does.

And so, of what unusual value is a "natural" cosmetic? Some interesting comments on these cosmetics have been made by a marketing specialist, Dr. Ernest Dichter, who heads the Institute for Motivational Research. The Institute seeks the psychological and sociological reasons why people buy the things they do.

Women who buy these cosmetics, he says, are trying— perhaps not quite consciously—to retrieve youth, to "counteract defloration and bring back virginity." Also, they are resisting the demands (presumably in advertising) of the Establishment that they buy traditional cosmetics. Thus they determine to use either a "natural" cosmetic or nothing. By using the "natural" types, says Dr. Dichter, they satisfy their psychological needs. He might also have said that thereby they fall into a trap of their own choosing, rather than having one dictated to them.

The sellers of "natural" cosmetics shrewdly make no bold claims in their advertising—not directly, anyway. They simply nudge the mind of the prospective buyer, quite subtly, in the direction of such highly acceptable concepts as "purity," "ecology," and "environment" and depend upon the process of mental association to take over from there.

Deodorants and Antiperspirants

The term "perspiration odor" is misleading. As I mentioned earlier, recent research has shown that perspiration itself is odorless. What produces the odor is the ever-present bacteria that seek out and thrive in perspiration-moist body areas such as the armpits and the genital and anal region.

You may observe that children in the prepuberty age seldom have body odors unless they go long unwashed. They have no underarm or genital hair to trap sweat. Nor do the odors trouble clean, older people, for their perspiring and hair growth have diminished.

That is why a fastidious woman would do well to keep her underarm hollows shaved. Though men are just as vulnerable to an odor problem, they don't usually bother with underarm shaving.

As we have seen, there are two kinds of sweating; they occur in different body areas although in some places they overlap. The kind caused by heat alone does not usually create much odor. But the sweat released by anxiety or nervous tension—seen on the forehead, palms of the hands, and soles of the feet—does bring on the problem.

The most effective prevention of body odor is among history's worst-kept secrets: proper and frequent bathing, daily changes of undergarments, regularly cleaned outer garments, and, advisedly, a daily change of shoes.

If ordinary soaps do not handle your ordinary perspiration, use an antiseptic soap. If something still stronger is needed, switch to one of the modern deodorant soaps. Even after bathing, small traces of antiseptic remain on the skin and repeated use builds up their effect. It should be emphasized, though, that the anti-bacterial action of an antiperspirant or a deodorant that contains an antiseptic, as many do, leaves the skin better protected than the antiseptic soap does. Still, soap-and-water bathing remains absolutely indispensable.

Avoid a deodorant claiming to contain antibiotics. The danger is that it actually may. Antibiotics are tricky even under close medical supervision and can sensitize the skin or produce allergic reactions. Besides, a bacterial organism will in time learn how to handle a specific antibiotic and will no longer be affected by it. Some deodorants are nothing but perfume, and can be worse than nothing because they give the user a feeling that bathing has become less important.

If you use an antiperspirant, a deodorant isn't necessary. The antiperspirant alone is enough, because it has everything the deodorant has, plus merits of its own. Antiperspirants usually contain aluminum chlorhydrate, though some contain zinc salts instead. In either case, the antiperspirant seems to have a real effect in reducing perspiration flow, though just how it does this is not clear. Also, the more it is used, the more effective it seems to become. It is unlikely to bring on a skin irritation. If it does, switch to a brand containing a different kind of aluminum salt, perhaps even zinc salt. The labels name the salts in the products. The labels don't always make it clear, however, whether the product is an antiperspirant or a deodorant.

Antiperspirants are more likely to be identified, or the label may use language suggesting that the product halts or checks perspiration. (It can never really "halt" perspiration; at best it can only slow down the flow.)

When used in a freshly shaved armpit, antiperspirants can cause considerable burning or stinging. The discomfort can last through the night. Indeed, smarting often occurs when they are used on any wet skin area, even if it is not newly shaved. However, there are many antiperspirants on the market that only occasionally cause reactions.

The form of antiperspirant or deodorant to use—spray, cream, roll-on, stick, bottled—is a decision that should be made according to personal convenience. They all appear to be equally effective. However, note this about the spray types: they come in aerosol cans and almost any aerosol chemical presents a real danger if you get a lungful. To avoid it requires no special precautions. A quick squirt or two aimed into an armpit certainly seems to pose no inhalation hazard.

Skin Blemishes Need Not Show

A disfiguring skin blemish is hardly a social or occupational advantage, but no longer need a life be blighted by it. Sometimes, as in the case of scarring, minor surgery is a helpful solution. But it is not the answer to some unsightly birthmarks or to limited skin areas where too much pigmentation causes dark spots, or too little pigmentation whitish spots. The enlargement of small blood vessels just under the top layer of skin will appear as bright red blemishes; in that situation it should be determined whether there is evidence of some skin disease that should be treated at the source. Several diseases can cause this symptom.

It was some years ago that an able, intelligent young woman found it difficult to hold a job because of an unsightly blemish that ran from chin to forehead. Not one to yield to that plight, she got a chemist interested in perfecting a substance that would effectively mask her stigma. He succeeded, and the boon of masking cream was born. Physicians immediately became interested in it as a means of dissolving the mental agonies of patients similarly afflicted.

In masking creams there is a concentration of "covering" chemicals—zinc oxide, kaolin, or others. They are mixed with a base similar to that of ordinary cosmetic creams—various combinations of mineral oil, lanolin, paraffin, other oils or waxes; color is added in a wide range of shades. A masking cream is most effective when it covers a skin-level mark like a pigment spot or other discoloration, which includes most birthmarks. Even a regretted tattoo can be concealed. Raised or indented scars, too, will usually be moderately hidden by masking cream, including those left by burns, acne, or surgery.

Successful use depends on a choice of the exactly right color and practicing to perfection the art of application. The right color is the one most like that of the skin around the mark, and good application means covering the blemish with the cream and blending it into the clear skin beyond. If the cream must go into the undereye area, where there is normally a shadow, a "shading cream" is available for blending with the masking cream. If the masking cream must cover the bridge of the nose or base of the chin, a small bit of rouge over the cream will contribute to a natural appearance.

Small or temporary blemishes of many types are easily covered by a masking stick, which can also conceal undereye circles and the lines of an aging skin.

In a case of active acne, ordinary masking cream should not be used because of its oily ingredients; besides, it would keep the acne medication from contact with the skin. There are many fat-free and wax-free foundation lotions that can be used without harm by patients suffering from acne.

Enlarged Pores

No matter what the ads say, nothing will open or close enlarged pores. But the appearance of rough skin that they create can be minimized for short periods. There are three types of skin openings that are commonly called "pores." One releases perspiration, the second emits natural body oil (sebum), and the third is the surface opening of the hair follicle. The first two are invisible but the third can be seen and may become enlarged in adolescence. The condition is most often noted on nose, cheeks, and chin. A youngster with enlarged pores often has acne too, and in time is likely to outgrow both. But it is these cases that frequently recur after the age of forty. There seems to be a general tendency for oily skin and enlarged pores to go together.

The basic methods of handling enlarged pores are two-fold. The first is the use of a makeup base that will conceal the enlargements and give the skin a smooth appearance. Trials of different kinds of makeup will soon point to the type most effective for a specific skin. If the skin is also oily, a liquid base is better than a cream. As a rule, foundations with heavy bases will not be as effective as those with light or medium covering ability.

The second way of dealing with enlarged pores is the use of an exfoliating lotion, which can be applied by the patient. The effect is to remove the outer layer of the skin, thus making the pores seem less prominent.

A simple astringent will create a mild irritation that causes the skin to swell slightly, thus making the enlarged pores less evident. One of the best such astringents is ordinary, low-priced witch hazel; plain rubbing alcohol is about as good. But some find these too harsh for regular use and resort to astringent cosmetic products, which are usually built on very simple formulas—a minimum of 35 percent alcohol (it should have no less), water, perfume, and a coloring agent. It may also contain zinc or aluminum salts, menthol, or allantoin. Astringents should be used in moderation and use should be stopped if inflammation or unusual redness appears.

Many preparations sold as "skin toner" or "skin freshener" are only weak astringents, but they do make the skin feel better and are useful where the stronger astringents are objectionable.

Cosmetics and Teen-agers

It is estimated that about 75 percent of young girls today begin to use lipstick by the age of fourteen, and nail polish much earlier. Since lipstick cannot be used secretly, most girls' parents obviously consent to their daughters' wearing makeup. My advice to the minority of dissenting parents can be summed up in the old proverb: if you can't lick 'em, join 'em. The awakening of an interest in makeup can be turned to an actual advantage in the daughter-rearing process.

After all, a youngster's use of cosmetics is not, as a rule, physically harmful. And makeup, wisely used, can do much to make a girl look and *feel* prettier by emphasizing her own special brand of good looks. As regards to the question of taste, the main point is that a girl today—especially a young girl—should seek a fresh, natural beauty and avoid a flashy, obviously "made up" look. This means that the knowing teen-ager who uses cosmetics will use them sparingly.

When a mother agrees—whether gladly or with a certain

sense of regretful resignation—that her young daughter may start wearing makeup, she should seize the opportunity to start her off, right from the beginning, with a sane and sensible understanding of the subject. A parent's counsel, which she should state clearly, might run something like this:

"If you're going to start using cosmetics, you should first know what they're for. They are intended to make your features look a little better than they really are—though not much. If moderate use doesn't bring about the miracle you want, increasing the dose will only make matters worse. With each type of cosmetic there comes a point of greatest benefit, and if you will watch carefully you will learn by experience where that point is.

"What's even more important is that the use of cosmetics is only one part—and a minor part—of looking your prettiest. They're a lot less important to beauty than a healthy body and a healthy skin are, because it is these that give you a glow that no cosmetics can replace. Personal cleanliness, as a matter of never-skipped routine, comes first. Cosmetics should be applied on a clean skin."

Too many parents overlook the definite benefits that can be associated with a girl's natural interest in cosmetics.

Not all youngsters clean hands and face before bedtime; to those who do not use cosmetics, the necessity for it can seem pretty remote. But the young teen-ager who must remove the day's makeup will do it with care, using soap and water or a cleansing cream. By doing this she learns a hygienic measure that might otherwise be by-passed. It may be noted that a girl starting to use makeup also begins to give more attention to the mirror, which alerts her to the presence of skin disorders in their early stages. Being more appearance conscious than a nonuser of cosmetics, she is also more likely to take the necessary steps to correct any skin problem whose sysmptoms she detects.

Beauty-awareness is a perpetual self-breeder. A teen-ager's concern with her face is an interest that quickly is extended to other parts of the body. She develops a livelier respect for regular and frequent bathing. With that comes a rising preoccupation with routine shampooing as she becomes aware that nothing means so much to attractive hair. At about the same time she learns about the **reward**ing hair-brushing regimen—the traditional one hundred strokes are fine, but a somewhat less strenuous number will do. These all become lifelong habits. By encouraging them, a mother fulfills a basic obligation as a parent.

Feminine Hygiene Sprays

Recent years have seen the development of a number of so-called feminine hygiene deodorant sprays. Unfortunately, the risks involved in the use of these sprays more than outweigh their possible benefits. One of those risks is that the user will adopt the spray as a replacement for indispensable soap and water. A significant number of cases of vulvar irritation have been reported, and these have been linked with regular use of the spray. If soap and water are used daily there should be no odor problem. If one persists, a vaginal discharge may be present. See your doctor.

A real danger can arise if the feminine spray is used internally. It remains in contact with the delicate vaginal tissue for hours with little opportunity to evaporate or otherwise dissipate. There have been medical reports that these sprays, as well as antiseptic vaginal douches, can irritate the tissues.

Beauty: Is It a State of Mind?

In a mentally healthy woman, the quest for beauty is controlled, disciplined. When it becomes a main preoccupation of life, it's neurotic. At the outset of this chapter,

I suggested that beauty was more an inner quality than a condition of the skin. Over the years, I have heard a number of versions of an experiment that has more recently been described in a book, *Symbolic Interaction,* by I. G. Manis and B. N. Meltzner.

It was conceived by a group of psychology graduate students, who planned to seek successive dates with the most unlovely-looking girl at the university. When that was determined, they drew lots—the winner doomed to date her first. He did, and spent the evening commenting on her attractiveness. The process was repeated by other members of the experimental group, who kept stepping up the level of flattery. In the process, this dowdy girl became more appearance-conscious—her clothing and hair became more neatly kept; more important, her negative personality opened up and she became more agreeable, more companionable. The fourth student on the list to take up the dating chore actually enjoyed his evening with her. The last man on the list struck out badly: when he asked for his date, she had to tell him she was booked up well into the future!

Is there a message there for all women?

5

Skin and Hair Aids for Men

Men, as well as women, have long taken advantage of what might be called "cosmetic" preparations. Our forefathers attached no stigma to the use of wig powder, hair tonic, or moustache wax. "Hair restorers" remained popular, despite the fact that they invariably promised more than they delivered.

Today, however, we find a far wider range of skin and hair aids offered for male use only. Though few of these aids have yet met with really wide commercial success, their use is becoming increasingly popular with men. The trend seems to have started mainly among younger males and then to have spread to the younger-in-heart among the older generation. The older generation had its special motive, too. With the greater emphasis being placed today on youthfulness in the arts, the professions, and even conservative business, the prevailing "youth syndrome" can have a very practical effect on a man's job. (Increasingly, corporations boast publicly of "the youthfulness of our management team.") It seems only a natural development, therefore, that men are increasingly using the new preparations available to help them maintain a youthful appearance and healthy-looking skin.

These preparations serve mainly to moisturize the skin, to protect it from the sun, to soothe it after shaving, to deodorize the armpits, and to shampoo the hair. Products containing protein can be used to thicken the hair. Some men like to use a slightly perfumed soap for the bath or shower. I heartily endorse the use of these products to clean and protect the skin and hair, to impart a pleasant fragrance, and to prevent perspiration odor.

One of the earlier products to offer a cosmetic, appearance-altering effect to males was the descriptively named Man Tan, which dyes the skin to a synthetic tan. Several competitive products have appeared since Man Tan emerged on the suntan scene about 1960 with its promise of instant, painless bronzing. It delivered on that promise, too—and the user did not need an instant's exposure to the sun. The secret of this magical transformation is a chemical called dihydroxyacetone, which simply dyes one's exterior. Unlike a real tan, it gives the skin no protection against sunburn. Some of these preparations, however, have since been vastly improved by adding a sunscreening ingredient. The sun stick and after-sun balms may be found helpful. We'll discuss the effects of the sun on the skin—and how to minimize them—more fully in Chapter 8.

The selling of men's skin and hair aids has become a burgeoning business. Two major cosmetic companies specialize in the production and distribution of a complete line of preparations to meet every need from head to toe. Male-type colognes and perfumes have been formulated with fragrances that are believed to be appealing to men (and to women too) without impairing masculinity. They come in both regular and spray form.

In the shaving department, besides the usual lathers, after-shave lotions, and talcums, there are preblade softeners for thick beards, preelectric shaver conditioners, after-shave balms to soothe the abraded skin, and tan like balms.

A special emollient cream for use after shaving is just as helpful for men as it is for their wives. In shaving, the razor removes a microscopic layer of skin, the top section of the "horny layer," which is hard and protective. It thereby exposes a softer, slightly more vulnerable layer that remains raw for a few hours. An after-shave lotion usually contains alcohol, which is an antiseptic but may also act as a further irritant especially to dry skins. A workable compromise is to apply the after-shave lotion, remove it quickly with a clean tissue, and then cover the skin with the soothing, softening, emollient cream. The absorbent type leaves no visible trace of its use. It is especially useful for a skin that is dry or beginning to show lines.

Other products for the face include a facial cleansing bar, a conditioning cream, a facial massage cream, a wrinkle cream, and bronzing cream or "bronzers" to impart a darker tone to the skin and simulate tanning.

New products marketed for the body area include an after-shower body rub, cooling spray, cooling foot spray, and a cologne deodorant spray.

Among the preparations available to help keep your hair and scalp clean, fresh, and healthy are shampoos for dry, regular, and oily hair; balsam protein shampoo, hair sprays, hair and scalp conditioners, and antidandruff hair dressings.

These and other special preparations for men can make the morning toilet pleasanter, leave your skin looking fresher and more youthful all day, enhance your sex appeal, and brace your ego as well as your skin.

In my dermatology practice I have been noticing two other areas of increasing cosmetic concern on the part of men. They are now less inclined to ignore residual facial scarring of early acne—which men once tended to believe lent them a quality of rugged masculinity—and they are increasingly interested in the process of dermabrasion, a technique that minimizes the scarring and sometimes can eradicate it entirely.

Others come in, in growing number, with a view to benefiting from the most modern *scientific*—I emphasize the word—findings regarding baldness, and they show a special interest in the process of hair transplanting. It is a lengthy, costly, and not entirely painless process, but their raised cosmetic goals have left men more willing to make the required sacrifices.

Shortly before the magazine *Look* expired, it carried an interesting story about cosmetic surgery, with some specific attention to its appeal to men. The article told of a prominent cosmetic surgeon in California who had his own receding hairline corrected by a colleague through hair transplants, then proceeded to do the same for his own brother.

Among men, the article reported on the basis of the experience of a number of cosmetic surgeons, the most sought-after operation was the face-lift, which most people believe to be a purely female recourse. While this is a procedure resorted to by older people, many middle-aged and even young men submit to corrective operations to improve the symmetry of their features or for other facial conditions that are less than dreadful.

The male, too, has been liberated, and today be can suit his own inclinations in buying and using cosmetic products to enhance his ego.

6

Cosmetic Dermatitis

If you are an average user of cosmetics, there is almost no cosmetic made today that will give offense to your skin. But a problem does arise when an average user ceases, for some unpredictable reason, to be average.

Before a new cosmetic product of any reputable manufacturer has reached its first store counter, the company's chemists and dermatologists have probably applied every known practical, reasonable test to insure the buyer's safety. But they could not have taken into account some factor whose potential adverse effect on *some* skins was unknown and, at the time, unknowable.

Just how many people, or what part of the total population, may be visibly sensitive to cosmetics is largely unknown. No sponsor has come along to finance the broadscale study needed; nor, probably, would there be enough volunteers to take part in a project of skin-testing that would reward them neither with adequate payment in coin nor with a sense of having contributed something truly vital to mankind. Making lipstick safe for users just doesn't seem that earthshaking.

However, two fairly large-scale tests conducted over a period of about thirty years have suggested that a very small percentage of the total population may be troubled by one cosmetic or another.

Broadly, the term dermatitis applies to any skin inflammation. There are many forms of dermatitis, caused by any of thousands of substances, singly or in combinations. Tracing and identifying these substances turns the doctor—be he general practitioner, dermatologist, or allergist—into a detective and the search can bring him to his wits' end. Often he must probe without much help from the patient, who is wholly without the resources to suggest any useful clue.

The frequent difficulty in zeroing in on the basic cause is that the culprit substance may be something seemingly innocent, apparently above suspicion. It could be as bland as talcum powder, as refreshing as toothpaste, as wholesome as buttermilk. It would never occur to a patient to mention any of these to a doctor looking for a "villain."

Medical lore tells of the dermatologist who was nearly distraught trying to find what substance in his patient's lipstick was causing her lips to swell, crack, and scale. It took months of testing, quizzing, and speculating before he came up with the answer—her boyfriend's moustache wax! An equally baffling case is recorded of a young man with a facial eruption. It took long and arduous grilling to establish Important Fact No. 1. His eruptions always came after an evening out with his girl friend. With that clue, the investigation proceeded the hard way, leading to the ultimate finding that the young man enjoyed nuzzling her beautiful red hair and that something in her hair rinse had sensitized him.

The main point here is that you may react painfully to *someone else's cosmetic.*

A Choice of Irritants

There are two general types of skin irritants: a primary irritant, which directly outrages the skin—almost any skin —by mere contact (hence "contact dermatitis"), causing redness, swelling, and pain, and a sensitizer, which sets up an allergic reaction after repeated contacts.

Primary Irritants: These are endless in number and variety. A woman is exposed to many each day—soaps, detergents, bleaches, cleaning fluids, scouring powders. The aluminum salts in her antiperspirant may be one, but it is her kitchen that has so many primary irritants that it has inspired the inclusive diagnostic term "housewives' dermatitis." A homemaker's hands may make contact with soap or detergent above a score of times a day.

If your hands get into trouble and develop red, irritated skin, the most sensible first step is to take each household cleaning product in turn and abandon its use for five or six days. If the objectionable condition clears up, you've solved your problem. As a substitute for the troublesome product, experiment until you've found one that will do the same household job without harmful effect to your skin. Most laundry bleaches, all of which are virtually identical, contain 5 or 6 percent of chlorine. Most scouring powders contain ammonia or potash. All these ingredients may act as irritants.

In any case, rubber or synthetic gloves are a good safeguard, especially if worn with a pair of thin cotton gloves under them.

Allergic Irritants: If, however, a skin reaction from a cosmetic is allergic in origin, the remedy is less simple. There is no telling in advance what may bring it on. Who could have predicted the consequences of the moustache wax or hair rinse?

Here is the root of the problem: repeated exposure to many types of bacteria may in time make one immune to them. But in the case of an allergy, the opposite is true—the more often we are exposed to a specific allergen (the basic substance to which an individual's skin reacts), the more sensitive we become to it.

Why some people react violently to a specific allergen, some mildly, and most of us not at all is anything but clear. Since certain allergies seem to run in families, heredity is often a factor. The entire subject is exposed in greater detail in Chapter 11, on allergy.

That the cause of a specific ailment is unknown does not mean we are helpless in coping with it. Fortunately, a great many diseases and disorders can be accurately diagnosed and successfully treated even though medical science is still far from knowing their causes.

Sensitizers: In many years of dermatologic practice I have investigated thousands of cases of cosmetic dermatitis caused by either an allergen or direct chemical assault. The chemical type is handled more easily, but I have observed that the allergy types occur mostly in patients who already have a history of allergy, not necessarily involving cosmetics. If your skin has in the past reacted to any substance at all, you should remain especially alert for eruptions from other causes.

A number of dermatologists have carefully catalogued cosmetic reactions of their patients and have listed them in the order of their frequency—in short, the cosmetic that most often causes trouble, then the one second in frequency, and so on. That their lists do not exactly correspond in order of frequency—though they are essentially not too different—may be due to the fact that these physicians practice in different parts of the country with differences in the patterns of product use, humidity, and climate.

I have my own catalogue of cosmetic hazards, compiled over a number of years. The list relates only to allergic reactions to cosmetics most often encountered, but I must point out that none of the products made the list because it was in any way "impure." These cosmetics will not trouble the vast majority of users, and an individual sensitive to one or more of them will not necessarily be sensitive to all. The purpose of specifying the range is to help those afflicted to narrow down more quickly the search for the culprit product.

Therefore, in a general, if not aways precise, order of their hazard, the cosmetics to watch in use are:

Nail polish
Lipstick
Hair dyes and bleaches
Deodorants and antiperspirants
Perfumes
Nail conditioners
Depilatories (hair removers)
Permanent waving materials
Hair-straightening products
Bleaching creams (especially with hydroquinone; see label)
Face and body creams with lanolin or perfumes
Suntanning lotions
Soaps with such photosensitizing agents as halogenated salicylanilides, usually advertised as deodorant soaps (after use, skin exposed to the sun *may* develop a rash)

There have also been more recent reports of allergic reactions traced to preservatives used in cosmetics.

How Cosmetic Problems Show Up

For those who do find themselves with a skin problem that may be related to cosmetics, this guide should help to run it down:

Nail polish dermatitis is becoming more frequent. The polish may cause a rash around the fingernails, of course, but also on eyelids, neck, chest, or any other part of the body that is touched or scratched with the polished nails. The allergen at fault is usually a specific resin in the polish (arylsulfonamide).

Lipstick often causes cosmetic dermatitis, and the alert user is usually able to make a correct diagnosis herself. There is burning, irritation, and sometimes swelling of the mucous membranes of the lips. Now that the "permanent" lipsticks are used less often, the condition is becoming less common. To achieve its greater durability, the product contains fluorescent dyes that may sensitize the lips. However, the fluorescent materials have in some instances been replaced by other chemicals that provide good staining in a wide range of colors. Lipstick dermatitis is diminishing also because of greater purification of some ingredients that formerly caused trouble.

Hair dye dermatitis has also become less common, but still occurs frequently. It is usually a reaction to a dye ingredient known as paraphenylenediamine. This dermatitis would be seen less if hairdressers applied a simple patch test twenty-four to forty-eight hours before treatment. The test uses a small sample of the dye substance, applied to the skin. If the test shows sensitivity to the dye, it may not be used. Problems arise because hairdressers often by-pass the test and use the dye anyway. An allergic reaction to a hair dye may come within a few hours; it will develop fully within a day or two at most. The scalp reacts severely, with redness, irritation, swelling, and perhaps seepage. The face, ears, and neck may also become involved. The eyelids can become quite puffy and swollen; sometimes the eyes will be completely closed.

Bleaching, too, can cause an identical reaction, most likely due to the peroxide and ammonia persulfate in the bleach. I have treated many hairdressers who have developed a contact dermatitis on the hands from repeated exposures to bleaches and dyes. Their affliction is further aggravated by detergents in the shampoos they handle. To a hairdresser this sort of sensitivity often means a forced change of trade.

Antiperspirant, if used frequently, can result in a dermatitis in the armpit hollow. It is due mainly to the product's aluminum compounds, especially aluminum chlorhydrate. The armpit perspiration seems to dissolve the aluminum compound and spread it through the armpit, causing an astringent action in the outer layers of the skin. Curiously, the deepest part of the armpit seems unaffected. However, this reaction vanishes quite soon after the use of the antiperspirant is discontinued. A deodorant also may cause a dermatitis, usually triggered by an antiseptic that it contains, such as hexachlorophene, or an antibiotic like neomycin.

Perfumes very often touch off a dermatitis, usually because of the process known as photosensitization. This means that when the sun hits the perfume a skin reaction results (some chemicals not found in perfumes produce a similar reaction). Thus moisturizing hand or body creams that contain perfume, as many of them do, also can mean trouble. With long, direct use of perfume—usually applied behind the ears or around the neck—exposure to sunlight may cause a brownish pigmentation to develop at those sites. This discoloration will take the shape of a hanging drop of fluid and is known as Berloque (or Berlock) dermatitis. Its fundamental cause is an essence, oil of bergamot, which is used in perfume. This oil is an ingredient of a very popular perfume. In hypoallergenic cosmetic products (made to be relatively free of possible allergens), perfume is strictly excluded. The pigmentation caused by perfume dermatitis often is permanent; its visibility may be somewhat reduced by bleaching cream.

Nail conditioners have been known to cause nail damage to an alarming extent. The fault lies with a basecoat developed some years ago for application to the nail to make the later coat of final polish more durable. It was found that a formaldehyde resin in these conditioners was causing discoloration, hemorrhaging, pus formation, and darkening under the nail plate. Packagers of such products sometimes have the grace to add a label instruction warning the user to protect the nail plate from injury by using a shield around the soft tissue and cuticle when applying the conditioner. It is vexing that patch tests often do not help in diagnosing this type of dermatitis.

Depilatories, for their active ingredient, often rely upon a rather harsh chemical, calcium thioglycolate, which dissolves and decomposes the hair shaft. There is often a reaction in the skin tissues around the hair shaft, especially on the face, although many depilatories are claimed in their advertising to be gentle enough for safe use on the face. Still, a depilatory must have a certain degree of chemical harshness if it is going to remove hair; it does not matter what part of the body is involved because the percentage of calcium thioglycolate is not changed for different parts of the body. A reaction to this type of depilatory is probably not allergic, but primary—that is, caused directly by a chemical attack on the skin.

Permanent waving and *hair straightening,* though they seek opposite results, actually depend upon the same basic chemical ingredient—the alkaline thioglycolate used in depilatories. It causes the hair to straighten temporarily, but if a wave is the desired end, further steps are then taken. The most common complaint following use of a thioglycolate compound for these purposes is that the hair breaks and splits. If the chemical is not properly neutralized, as directed on the label, the breakage can be severe. I have seen many cases of hair damage caused by both straighteners and wavers, though the straighteners usually have a rougher time of it. This sort of complaint reached its

peak at the height of the straight-hair fad among both
sexes. A dermatitis usually accompanies the hair breakage;
there is scalp inflammation with related scaling, reddening,
and swelling around the hair follicles, as well as some hair
loss. As a result, the thioglycolate portion of some straighteners has been reduced; while they do a less effective
straightening job, they also cause less hair and scalp
damage.

Bleaching creams have risen in use in recent years because of an increase in the occurrence of hyperpigmentation of the face—dark pigmented spots or areas larger than
mere spots. There are several possible reasons for the pigmentation increase. There is now greater use of perfumes
and antiseptics—either alone or as ingredients of other
products applied to the skin—which cause a skin reaction
when exposed to the sun (photosensitivity). Also, it has
often been reported that regular use of contraceptive pills
can cause such skin discolorations (see Chapter 15, on the
Pill). And finally, many eager sun worshipers have found
that the coming of winter has not dissolved their suntans
entirely, but has left some of it in the form of ugly, dark
spots. For many years ammoniated mercury was used to
bleach out such spots, but it has more recently been replaced by some relatives of the hydroquinone family, which
not only bleach but also help to suppress excessive pigmentation. These chemicals, to be effective, require extended use, which in turn also raises a danger of contact
dermatitis.

Face creams or *body creams* can also produce a contact
dermatitis, which may arise from an ingredient such as
perfume, lanolin, or propylene glycol. For most of us,
lanolin, the oil taken from a sheep's wool, can be both
boon and balm as the substance most like the human
body's natural oil. Some people's skin, however, reacts

poorly to it, as patch testing will prove. In a large New York clinic, only a small percentage of 1,500 patients tested for lanolin reactions proved to be susceptible. Used in many cosmetics, propylene glycol is usually inoffensive but is an allergen to some skins. It is becoming a common glycerin substitute, which means it is coming into contact with more people's skin. In its favor are its antibacterial action and its ability to combine other elements in a cosmetic formula.

Suntanning and *sunscreening lotions,* while designed to prevent painful skin damage, are also capable of causing eruptions. When they do, the source of damage is likely to be their perfume or a sunscreening agent in the form of a para-aminobenzoic acid. A sunscreening or sun-blocking agent is the most important ingredient in a suntan lotion, which is a must for people with unusual sun sensitivity. One of the most effective sunscreens is the benzophenone referred to as a "light absorber." Anyone who develops a severe reaction to this type of lotion should not blame the product. The benzophenone may have sensitized the user to it when the skin was exposed to the sun—another example of photosensitivity. A skin discoloration may result, but an emollient should clear that up in time.

Soaps can cause a skin eruption, especially dermatitis of the hands—the so-called housewives' eczema. The alkali in the soap is the usual cause. The skin may react directly to contact with the soap or to the soap's action in defatting the skin of its natural oils. Or it may be that the soap is too alkaline and has shifted the skin's normal acid/alkali (pH) balance, which must always favor the acid side for good skin health; the favorable balance is called the "acid mantle." The critical acid mantle stops working for you when the alkali becomes dominant in the skin balance. The relatively recent introduction of premium-price deodorant soaps has brought some problems. Many skin reactions have been traced to them, and more specifically to their antiseptic ingredients. An alert British physician was first to report an increase of dermatitis of the hands and face during the summer months; many patch tests he performed led him to the antiseptic soaps.

How to Handle Cosmetic Dermatitis

Luckily, ending most outbreaks of cosmetic dermatitis is relatively simple, whether the root of the problem is physical contact with a suspected cosmetic or an allergy that it has set up. These are the steps to be taken, either together or in sequence:

1. Simply stop using the suspected cosmetic. If there is no improvement in a few days, eliminate Cosmetic Suspect No. 2, then No. 3, and so on.

2. Meanwhile, for as long as the skin misbehaves, apply antiseptic compresses to the afflicted area (s), preferably Burow's solution.

3. If the condition still persists, taking an antihistamine would be helpful, but would require a prescription. Still, at that point you should be seeing a doctor anyway.

4. If irregular skin discolorations have appeared, and refuse to leave after the eruptions have gone, try an emollient or bleach cream. If that doesn't help in a reasonable time, go back to Step 3 above—the doctor.

Listed in Appendix I are cosmetic products most often associated with allergy, together with the ingredient in each that is most likely the basic cause of the problem. The chemical names will probably be unfamiliar, but if any of them proves to be a special nemesis of yours, memorize it—or as many as you need. For example, if you find yourself sensitive to a nail conditioner, you must begin to avoid its chief allergen, formaldehyde. Formaldehyde is found not

only in cosmetics but also in antiseptics and some household cleansers, and in any form can bring you fresh woe.
Become, therefore, a more regular label-reader. It will be
rewarding.

You will notice that some types of cosmetics may contain
more than one potential allergen. If you have discovered
the type of cosmetic that is making life difficult for you and
it contains more than one of these allergens, your next step
is to experiment with another brand containing only one
of these troublemakers. If you do get it narrowed down that
far, toss that last brand into the disposal and get a brand
that contains none of them. If you were to do that in the
first place without experimenting, you would probably
never know which one your allergen was.

Frequently it is advisable to consult a dermatologist and
have him patch-test you with each of your cosmetics to find
the offending agent. Once it's found, you can substitute
another cosmetic and all will be well.

7

Your Skin and Your Diet

This is perhaps the most important chapter in this book. Many years ago, a sage scientist and philosopher said, "The skin is the mirror of the body," meaning that frequently when a body is disordered or diseased there are changes in the skin. For example, hepatitis, a disease of the liver, causes yellowing of the skin and eyeballs, as in jaundice. Pellagra, due to deficiency in Vitamin B, causes pigmentation and roughness of the exposed dermal areas. Scurvy, a deficiency of Vitamin C, causes ecchymosis, a bruising of the skin and bleeding from the gums.

The skin and the hair, as integral parts of the human body, require adequate nutrition. This must be supplied through the circulation and lymph vessels to help the skin and its appendages revitalize themselves by replacing the parts that have been worn out.

The small capillaries in the skin are fed from the arterial part of the circulatory system and the blood then returns to the heart through the venous system.

Since nourishment for the skin is provided from the blood stream, the reader must realize that penetration by substances from the outside of the skin is minimal. Certain chemicals may be able to enter the blood stream from the outside, particularly through the openings of the hair follicles and pores. Some of these materials are hormones, steroids, and vitamins. These medications are usually dispersed in vehicles prescribed by physicians. They usually contain dimethyl sulfoxide and dimethyl acetamide.

Nutrition is, therefore, as essential for skin function as for any other part of the body. A healthy skin is well nourished, though it should also be well cared for externally by the methods described elsewhere in this book.

The cells of the cutaneous tissues need proteins to manufacture new cells, carbohydrates for energy, fats for energy and absorption of fat-soluble vitamins, and vitamins and minerals for specialized functions. Since modern processing of foods usually reduces their natural amounts of vitamins, trace minerals, and enzymes, supplements may be necessary.

In his excellent book *Nutrition Against Disease,* Dr. Roger J. Williams, the noted biochemist, writes: "The most basic weapons against disease are those most ignored by modern medicine; the numerous nutrients that the cells of our body need: all amino acids, all minerals, trace elements, about fifteen vitamins, probably many other coenzymes, nutrilites, and metabolites."

In another fine book, *Nutrition in a Nut Shell,* Dr. Williams points out: "The skin is a region which is known to be affected by many nutritional lacks. Scarcely a deficiency exists which does not manifest itself by pathological changes in the skin. This has been demonstrated particularly in animals, where it is possible to carry out conclusive experiments. There is evidence that acne, eczematous dermatitis, and even psoriasis (a condition which is almost by definition mysterious and incurable) may . . . have a nutritional origin."

Similarly, Dr. Anthony Domonkos, in an excellent textbook chapter on deficiency diseases, describes various skin disorders that he attributes to a lack of one or more dietary essentials.

Vital Food Elements

Let us review some of the most important food elements and see how their presence in or absence from the diet affects the body.

Vitamin A, found abundantly in butter and also present in fish and yellow fruits and vegetables, is important in many ways. A diet deficient in this vitamin may result in lowered resistance to infection; poor appetite and digestion; a dry, rough skin; an eye disease called xerophthalmia; and splotchy marks on the skin. To secure enough Vitamin A is not difficult as long as the diet is a varied one. Even if butter is eliminated completely, as it sometimes may be for weight reduction or other medical reasons, an occasional fish dish and the regular eating of yellow fruits and vegetables easily supply the daily requirement. Too much Vitamin A can also be dangerous. One of the symptoms of an excess can be the loss of hair.

Vitamin B is really a complex composition of different substances, including thiamine (B_1), riboflavin (B_2), niacin or nicotinic acid (which has nothing at all to do with the nicotine in tobacco, despite the similarity of names), pyridoxine (B_6), Vitamin B_{12} and others. Vitamin B_{12} is essential for the prevention of anemia and for the formation of protein in the body, and it also aids in the conversion of carbohydrates into fat.

Deficiencies in the various components of the Vitamin B complex can cause a variety of ailments, including many affecting the skin. Riboflavin deficiency, for example, is primarily manifested by impaired vision and itching, and burning sensations of the eyes, but also in scaling and cracking of the skin, especially on the lips. Pantothenic acid, also in the Vitamin B group, is believed to be essential for maintaining hair color, and graying hair (actually the turning of some hairs white, producing the gray effect) has been associated with a pantothenic acid deficiency. The same is true of para-aminobenzoic acid, still another member of the B complex. In studies with rats, it was found that black hair turned gray when para-aminobenzoic acid was withheld from the diet, and turned black again when it was restored. Attempts to duplicate these effects in human beings, however, have not been successful. There is no reliable evidence that this substance will restore color to gray human hair.

Nicotinic acid (niacin), also belonging to the B complex, is sometimes called the P-P (for "pellagra preventing") factor. Pellagra, a disease associated with malnutrition, is marked by crusted skin rashes as well as intestinal and mental disorders. Niacin is also an excellent dilator of the blood vessels. Niacin and its ester niacinamide are being used in the United States for treatment of mental disorders in massive doses of 1,000 milligrams daily in combination with 1,000 milligrams of Vitamin C. I have seen in my office several patients under the care of psychiatrists whose acne has improved under this regimen in conjunction with local treatment.

Vitamin C, also known as ascorbic acid, is the scurvy-preventing factor. Long before the word "vitamin" was coined, it was observed that sailors on long voyages could avoid scurvy if lime juice were a regular part of the diet, and British sailors are still called "limeys" in the United States because of the daily ration of lime juice they received. Scurvy is marked by bleeding gums and bloody diarrhea as well as by red spots on the skin around hair follicles and sweat pores. Oranges and lemons also provide Vitamin C, as do berries, peppers, and uncooked cabbage.

Incidentally, Dr. Linus Pauling, the Nobel Prize winner, in his book, *Vitamin C and the Common Cold*, extolls the use of high doses of Vitamin C for the prevention of colds. It is difficult, however, to carry out scientific studies to corroborate his theories.

Vitamin D helps prevent rickets, a disease that leaves bones weak and deformed. Cod-liver oil is rich in Vitamin

D. Its beneficial effect can be duplicated by exposing the skin to ultraviolet rays. A child with rickets, given adequate supplies of calcium and phosphorus, will improve just as well under exposure to natural ultraviolet light as to Vitamin D given internally.

Vitamin E is found in so many foods that its role is not well understood; there's very little opportunity to observe what deficiencies would result if a person were deprived of it for a long period of time. However, it has been found useful in large doses in helping the healing of various skin and vascular diseases, including ulcers of the skin, and is believed to be important in the function of the corium, or true skin.

Though it has become a popularly used vitamin, *Vitamin E* remains controversial. Its active ingredient is alpha-tocopherol. It is found in wheat germ oil, rice germ, cottonseed, green leafy vegetables, nuts, salad oils, and margarine. It is believed to prevent Vitamin A from being destroyed in the intestinal tract, protects the red blood cells from destruction, and has been used in skin diseases affecting deep cutaneous tissues. In a survey I conducted, topical use of highly concentrated Vitamin E has improved roughness and lines in the skin.

Amino acids are essential for cell reproduction and body health. They are usually secured from animal or vegetable products. Meats, milk, casein, various seeds, and beans, especially soy beans, contain large quantities of amino acids. There are twenty-six amino acids contained in food protein, eight of which are essential, and the body is not capable of synthesizing them. They are tryptophan, phenylalanine, lysine, threonine, methionine, leucine, isoleucine, and valine. Without these, life cannot exist. Two others, histidine and arginine, are semiessential in that they are not synthesized in adequate amounts during growth.

A detailed chart of minerals and vitamins, their values in the diet, and their sources, will be found in Appendix II.

Your Skin Reflects Your Diet

There are, as can be gathered from these brief comments, several ways of inviting skin manifestations through improper diet. Yet it is hardly necessary for everyone to memorize the minimum daily requirements for each vitamin to be sure he eats enough to satisfy each requirement every day. As a matter of fact, the vitamin-deficiency diseases are quite rare nowadays in countries where a wide variety of nourishing foods are available all year round. We see far more skin troubles among overweight people than among the slim, and I therefore advise my patients to take off excess weight and try to keep it off. One of the easiest ways in the world to gain unnecessary pounds, believe it or not, is to fret over whether you've had enough of a given vitamin, fat, protein, or starch on a given day, and then eat something you don't need "just to be on the safe side."

Eating too much isn't playing safe at all, with respect to the skin or any other aspect of health. We know that overweight people have a lower life expectancy than those of normal build, being more susceptible to heart disease, diabetes, and a host of other ills. As far as the skin is concerned, heavy people are prone to have the most trouble, partly because they chafe themselves where skin gathers in folds, partly because they must perspire more than those of lighter build, and partly because the circulatory system must do much work to serve the excess poundage, and can't concentrate on its regular jobs, one of which is the supplying of nutrients to the skin.

A sound diet for a healthy skin should consist of a selective amount of proteins; lean meats; milk; poultry; fish (shellfish, such as lobster, shrimp, and clams, not more than once every two weeks because of their high iodine and cholesterol content, and sea pollutants); nonspicy cheese, such as cottage, cream, Cheddar, and Gruyère; and fats, particularly such unsaturated fats as are contained in corn oil, peanut oil, sesame oil, and olive oil. There should be generous helpings of fruit, vegetables, and salads. Low-calorie salad dressings are preferred. Natural seasonings such as oregano, thyme, celery seed, chives, curry, garlic, ginger, nutmeg, paprika, sage, poppy seeds, and tarragon are preferred to salt.

The food should be cleansed to remove contaminants such as pesticides. Read the labels and reduce your intake of foods containing BHT, BHA, sodium nitrate, and emulsifiers which are used as fillers or stabilizers. By avoiding excess amounts of salt, sugar, and animal fats (cholesterol) you will add life to your years and years to your life. Eggs should be poached or boiled and eaten in moderation, especially in the older age group. The meals should be small and frequent, so as to permit easy assimilation and to avoid gastric discomfort. The skin will then receive the nutrients necessary for an attractive and healthy appearance, barring hormonal or metabolic diseases.

In caring for the skin, we must remember that a healthy skin is pleasing to the eye and that a woman can't be considered attractive or a man handsome if the skin is chafed, irritated, blemished, broken out, or discolored. But neither is a person of either sex very attractive when carrying around excess poundage. More important, I have noticed that overweight people, who have already lost some of their personal appeal by letting themselves get fat, are less inclined to care adequately for their skin, apparently feeling that their overall appearance is already below standard. In short, heavyweights develop a "What's the use?" attitude about their appearance and tend to neglect their skin as well as their general health. I much prefer to see a slim patient than a chubby one, simply because the former will be much more cooperative in carrying out treatment measures.

Where it is necessary to supplement the diet with additional vitamins—and let me emphasize again that this is necessary only for people who are not getting proper nutrition, such as those on crash diets or elderly people existing mostly on tea and toast—the recommended daily dosage range of ten basic vitamin supplements is as follows:

Vitamin A	5,000 International units
Vitamin B_1 (thiamine)	1.8–2.4 milligrams
Vitamin B_2 (riboflavin)	0.9–2.7 milligrams
Vitamin B_6 (pyridoxine)	1–3 milligrams
Vitamin B_{12}	2–10 milligrams
Vitamin C (ascorbic acid)	25–110 milligrams
Vitamin D	400 International units
Niacin (nicotinic acid)	12–20 milligrams
Pantothenic acid	5–10 milligrams
Folic acid	0.3 milligrams

Nowadays much emphasis is being placed on so-called natural or organic foods, as contrasted to synthetic foods, and there is an increased emphasis on vitamin intake, oral and local use of herbal applications, and intake of herbal teas and tinctures.

In this chapter I have attempted to describe the importance of a balanced diet, supplemented by adequate vitamins and trace minerals. Not only is skin and hair health improved through proper diet, but also normal body functions are protected. Medical supervision should always be maintained if skin disorders remain refractory in spite of balanced nutrition and vitamin intake.

8

The Sun Is Your Undoing

It was thirty years ago at this writing that a novel appeared and became quickly popular. It was *The Sun Is My Undoing* and I no longer remember the plot. But I recall the title every year, specifically every summer, and I am not sure the author, Margaret Steen, would have felt flattered to know what triggers my recollection of her poetic title. The stimulus is quite prosaic.

It is the procession of patients who come into my office with flaming, hurtful evidence that the sun has indeed left them undone—and, paradoxically, too well-done.

Sunburn is skin damage, and nearly always self-inflicted.

Everyone knows by now how it can be avoided—by gradual exposure that should normally be increased each day, until one develops a tan that gives reasonable protection from sunburn—though don't count on that protection too heavily.

If that were all there is to it, this chapter could end here and we could go on to something else. But for both the treatment and the avoidance of sunburn there are judgments that must be made and you will be able to make them more wisely if you know something about the sunburn-suntan process, the absolute rules that govern it, and, you may be pleased to know, some exceptions to those rules.

The Dangerous Sun

The villain of the plot is the sun itself—the warm, friendly, life-giving, treacherous and murderous sun. Choose the side you want to live with.

The sun is constantly bombarding us with rays of different kinds, but the atmosphere intercepts all but a small percentage of them. Of those that get through and make contact with the skin—which is the body's second barrier after the atmosphere—some are light rays, which become diffused and reflected and make it possible for us to see. Two others in the spectrum that are of prime importance to life are invisible to the eye. They are the infrared rays, which are hot and are used by the skin for warmth, and the ultraviolet rays, which convert the cholesterol and ergosterol in the skin to Vitamin D, a truly life-giving force. They confer other vital bodily benefits, too, but these ultraviolet rays *alone* cause the sunburn.

The sun's rays are measured in terms of their wavelengths, which are given places on the Angstrom scale, named after the scientist who devised it. The "shortest" of the rays reaching us are the ultraviolet, which fall in the range of 2,900 to 3,900 A (Angstrom).

But the sunburn rays are those in the range of 2,900 A to about 3,200 A; above that figure, the rays produce direct tanning, not burning. The idea, then, is to screen out the 2,900 A–3,200 A range and let the higher ones come through. That is what the so-called suntan creams and oils are all about. Actually, none of them has anything whatever to do with the tanning process, no matter what the claims may be; to be worth anything, they should screen out a large proportion of the burning ultraviolet rays, and nothing more than that should be expected of them.

Melanin—Nature's Defense Against Sunburn

Another unfounded notion persists; it is the belief that a

sunburn, in the healing process, is somehow converted into a suntan. The two are, in fact, quite unrelated and separate. What causes tanning is melanin, the pigment that determines the shade of your skin—your normal complexion shade. It lies at the bottom of the outer skin layer, the epidermis, and if the supply is abundant your skin will be darker than those who are shy of melanin, such as blonds, redheads, and, in general, people with blue eyes. Skins that are called black—though none ever gets that dark, really—have the greatest measure of melanin. An albino has almost none.

The dark melanin pigment is one of the major protectors against sunburn; thus, people with dark complexions are more or less immune to it. Scientists have determined that brunettes have more tolerance for ultraviolet rays than do blonds. A scientific method called Saldman's Sensometric Test has further shown that we react differently to the sun at different ages. The most *resistant* ages are from three and a half to five years, thirteen to seventeen, and fifty to sixty. The most *vulnerable ages* are, among children, from six to eight, among women, from twenty-five to thirty, and among men, from thirty to thirty-five.

Melanin is manufactured by cells called melanocytes, which lie in the bottom layer of the skin; for most of the year they live an easy existence, producing just enough melanin and sending it up to keep your complexion uniform. During the hot, sunshiny months, though, they're kept quite busy. When the ultraviolet rays penetrate the skin, the "longer" of them (above about 3,300 A) activate the melanin pigment near the surface and darken it. The "shorter" rays, however, pass through the skin and burn it in the process, causing redness and blistering. This warns the cells that things are getting pretty hot upstairs and they proceed at once to manufacture more pigment to be moved upward.

Within about two days the new dark pigment begins to

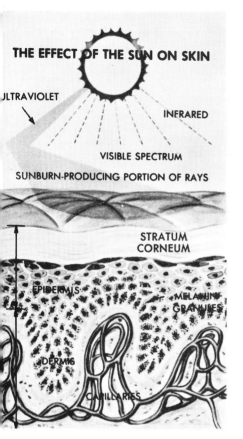

THE EFFECT OF THE SUN ON SKIN

ULTRAVIOLET

INFRARED

VISIBLE SPECTRUM

SUNBURN-PRODUCING PORTION OF RAYS

STRATUM CORNEUM

EPIDERMIS

MELANIN GRANULES

DERMIS

CAPILLARIES

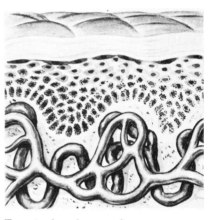

Twenty-four hours after exposure
of the skin to the sun,
the capillaries are dilated,
causing reddening.

One week after exposure—
the melanin granules are moving
into the stratum corneum,
which thickens to prevent
further burning.
(*DIAGRAMS COURTESY* TODAY'S HEALTH,
AMERICAN MEDICAL ASSOCIATION)

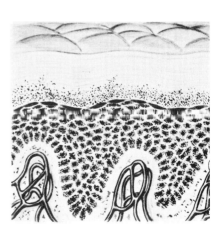

arrive where it's needed and the skin starts to darken, thereby minimizing the chance of further sunburn with the next exposure. In from five to seven days the tanning should be quite advanced, and further exposure should deepen it painlessly.

If there has also been significant sunburn, it should be diminishing as the tan comes in, although that is coincidental and not, as I have noted, cause-and-effect. You may have noticed in such a situation that there is a crossover point at which there are evidences of both redness and tanning at the same time.

How the Skin Heals Sunburn—at a Price

Sunburn is not unique among burns. Depending on its severity, the body responds just as it does to a burn caused by steam or hot grease. The skin shows erythema, or redness, the blood vessels swell, and fragile tissues break. If the burn is not too severe, the repair of the broken tissue begins in a few days; fluid is released from the damaged cells and inflamed blood vessels; in more serious cases the fluid forms in blisters on the surface and when they burst they peel from the outer layer. The dead and damaged cells slough off and are replaced by others that move up from below. However, they are somewhat harder and thicker than those that preceded them.

It is this new extra thickness of the outer skin that is thought to be at least as useful as melanin is in resisting further bouts of sunburn. While this process is beneficial to the immediate need, it is also an introduction to one of the long-range—and permanent—dangers of extended overexposure to the sun. More exposure means more hardening and thickening, and in time the skin becomes tough, leathery, dried, and usually blotched. Given enough time and exposure to the sun's flamethrower, the face can end up brown and corrugated. In the meantime, degenerative changes have been taking place in the skin's deeper layers and in the connective tissue, which lose their elasticity. By now, the wrinkles and grooves and ruts are largely irreversible. Proper and regular skin care thereafter might reduce the washboardy look somewhat, but not a great deal. To make the condition less visible only such dermatological techniques as dermabrasion or chemosurgery may be effective.

With more people now retiring to live in sunny or even semitropical climates, there are now more elderly folk who have time to spend soaking up sun. Often they develop wartlike pigmentation spots, either caused or aggravated by the sun. They are sometimes called liver spots but are in fact seborrheic keratodes or solar keratodes; light-skinned people are most susceptible to them.

Skin Cancer

The greatest hazard of long-term exposure to the sun, however, is skin cancer. The statistical evidence is overwhelming. This cancerous or precancerous condition was first related to the sun in the late nineteenth century by Dr. P. G. Unna of Germany. Among young sailors, he noted, the face, neck, hands, and the V on the upper chest, exposed by the sailor blouse, became ridged and leatherly while the skin elsewhere matured normally. Dr. Unna rejected a contention that wind and rain caused it, since sailors cover up in such weather. The sun alone, he insisted, was responsible for this condition, which he called "sailor's skin." It is also called "solar skin," or because farmers, too, are much exposed to the sun, "farmer's skin."

In the past few years there has been soaring evidence, even stronger than Dr. Unna's, of the skin's vulnerability to strong sunlight. The most compelling came from Dr. John M. Knox and associates at the Baylor University College of Medicine, Houston, Texas. They used a number of test subjects, both male and female prison volunteers, their ages ranging from twenty-five to seventy-six and their complexions from light blond to black. From each were taken three small samples of skin, *highly* exposed to the sun, *occasionally exposed,* and *never* exposed.

Findings under microscopic and other examinations were about as expected. *Heavily* exposed samples showed changes ranging from mild curling to significant damage that caused almost total loss of skin elasticity; as the outer layer became tough and leathery, layers below it became thinner and less able to receive supporting nutrients.

Samples of *occasionally* exposed skin showed much less damage, while the *unexposed* samples showed none at all. The experiments pointed up something else of interest; all skin samples from blacks, who seldom sunburn because of their increased melanin pigmentation, *showed no visible sun damage whatever.*

None of these disturbing consequences is likely to occur to people who spend summer weekends at the beach, even if they overdo the sunning somewhat. But those living in predominantly warm regions are by no means immune if they do not constantly take evasive action. A University of Chicago study showed that 90 percent of all skin cancers seen were on exposed parts of the body—face, neck, ears, even hands. In warmer parts of Australia, where the year offers eight sunny months, 20 percent of the average dermatologist's practice is devoted to treatment of skin cancers, a startling figure. Reports of that nature, though less radical, also come from the South and Southwest of the United States. Mountainous regions, too, show a high incidence of skin cancer—for which the scientific term is basal cell epithelioma—because there is less atmospheric interference offered to the ultraviolet rays; for another thing, there is less smog, which, whatever its other faults are, serves to block the ultraviolet rays, although ordinary fog and clouds do not.

Most skin cancers are treated successfully, but it's no fun.

It should be noted that skin cancer victims are largely fair-skinned. Even after you have acquired a deep tan, however, or if your skin tone is naturally rather dark, you are not immune to the increasing buildup of the hardening top layers of skin that, at the least, can cause wrinkling.

This build-up, which is called hyperkeratinization, is not restricted to the middle-aged and aged. It is a time bomb with a long fuse that can be lighted in the upper teens or early twenties. It has been widely observed in the medical literature that some sun-lovers at twenty already appear to be thirty, and at thirty appear to be forty. At 40—and my own observation confirms it—the heliophiles who began sun-worshiping at an early age may look like sixty!

Photosensitivity and Photoallergy

Unfortunately, there are two types of body responses to sunlight that will cause reactions varying in violence even when there is *no overexposure.*

The first condition is called *photosensitivity (photo* meaning light). It is caused not by an internal physical condition but by something taken internally or applied to the skin externally that finds sunlight disagreeable and reacts harshly to it. It can happen with relatively brief sun exposure soon after you have taken some drug such as an antibiotic, a tranquilizer, sedative, or diuretic. Or it may be provoked by a perfume, as described on page 92, by a cosmetic, or even by something within a suntan lotion itself. The symptoms are those of a sudden, violent sunburn —redness, inflammation, perhaps swelling.

The remedy is to get out of the sun quickly, and the surprise attack will probably subside shortly. If redness remains, an emollient cream should be used. Then try to determine which of the factors noted above may have been the one enraged by the sun so that you will avoid the combination in the future.

Photoallergy is a more serious matter. It means an essential intolerance of the sun, just as one may have an allergic intolerance of fish, dust, or plants. The visible reactions are an outbreak of a skin manifestation resembling hives, with attendant redness, swelling, temperature, perhaps nausea and other symptoms of severe sunburn. Here, again, it means getting out of the sun quickly, using emollient cream, and taking all the standard antisunburn measures. In addition, a doctor should be seen for counseling on how to avoid a recurrence, and the extent of the defense measures will depend upon the degree of sensitivity. If it is not very great, it might not be too chancy to resort to very brief, and frequent, exposures to build up a tolerance to sunlight. If that brings on no intolerable mischief, it may be advisable to take short sessions under an ultraviolet lamp during the winter months to build up a tolerance for the summer ahead.

Block That Sunburn!

Whatever the degree of solar hypersensitivity, a practical approach to the problem just before an unavoidable exposure is to cover all the parts that will be exposed with a *sunblock* cream. While a good *sunscreening* preparation will turn away from the skin a large proportion of the oncoming ultraviolet rays, a sunblock will filter out almost all of them, although the relatively few that come through may be enough to cause some minimal redness.

The sunblock preparation, incidentally, might be profitably used by people with normal sun reactions when they go to an area where the sunlight is especially intense. In such situations a sunscreen may not be enough, and the sunblock should be used the first two or three days to provide a gradual adjustment. I have found that idea to be prudent.

It is the sunscreen in cream or lotion form, however, that literally saves the hides of most of us in summer, and that means about 100 million of us. The first of these chemical defenses appeared commercially in 1928 as a standard, effective preventive remedy, offered as a replacement for a long, historic range of preventives and cures that neither prevented nor cured, but had nevertheless acquired large followings of loyal partisans, usually hereditary. Until then, one might be risking bodily harm to question aloud the true antisunburn qualities of mineral oil tinted with iodine, tea leaves, cold cream, cocoa butter, or any of scores of other "folk" remedies.

Mineral oil does nothing to retard sunburn, but it cannot be called harmless. As the sun reaches your oil-coated skin, the ultraviolet rays knife right through, but more than that, the mineral oil magnifies the rays just as a magnifying glass would and *multiplies* their potency. When mixed with vinegar and tannic acid, an old and popular combination, mineral oil isn't much better, although some derivatives of tannic acid have sunscreening properties.

Cocoa butter has had a following for some generations now, and in recent years has been used increasingly as an ingredient of sunscreen products. Its benefit, however, is as a moisturizer, for its sunscreening merits are negligible. There seems to be a misconception prevailing about cocoa butter. One arises from a confusion of the word with "coconut." Hawaiians use coconut oil before exposure to the sun, and it is assumed that Hawaiians are especially knowledgeable about such things. It's unlikely that they are, because coconut oil offers little or no screening, and Hawaiians, being dark-skinned, don't need much. Anyway, while cocoa butter will indeed help soften the skin and soothe a sunburn, it's very messy to use and will stain fabric. Besides, it is hard to apply and to remove.

Zinc oxide ointment often covers the noses of beach lifeguards. It blocks out the sun's rays quite well, but only if applied in a layer so thick that problems later arise in removing it. A commercial cream will work as well.

An Ounce of Prevention . . .

If we would look upon sunburn and its related consequences as a disease—as a painful, disabling illness, or at least, as serious skin damage—we would not be constantly challenging the sun to do its worst. But we are psychologically handicapped by a feeling that sunburn is only an uncomfortable means to a very desirable end—an alluring tan that suggests an exotic glow of health. And we are given to forgetting last summer's agony and the tearful vow, "Never again!"

So we get to the beach or the mountain lake just as soon as weather permits and we resume the cycle of folly. The fact is that on that first day, lying in the sun fifteen minutes on each side is quite enough; after that, the dose may be increased by five or ten minutes per side and stepped up by the same time interval for several days until the exposure is thirty or forty minutes per day per side. That would be a maximum daily dose of nearly an hour and a half after the tan arrives, which will surely meet all of your tanning needs. For small children, cut those dosages in half.

Instead of observing this prudent, disciplined course, people go to the beach, expose as much skin as possible, and lie there until the first redness appears. When it does, a delayed-action sunburn has already arrived—delayed until it really blossoms in from two to five hours.

Or, relaxed in the friendly warmth, the sunbather will fall asleep for an hour or so, and then the fat is literally in the fire. Having applied a sunscreen cream or lotion will help a good deal, but one application will not be good for an hour of intense sun, which will have dried up a large share of it. If one goes into the water for a brief swim, the sunscreen will be pretty well washed off. Then it should be renewed, the thicker the better. Contrary to a fairly widespread belief, the water does not retard the sunburning process; on the contrary, the bather takes not only the direct rays of the sun but also the rays reflected from the water.

When the Sun Is Closest

The number of minutes of exposure you can take at one sitting varies with several factors, as noted—natural complexion, degree of tanning already present, abnormal reactions, smog conditions, whether you're near reflective sand or water or on a rooftop. The season and other factors enter into it too. June 21 is the first day of summer, when the earth is nearest the sun; the danger is greatest that day, at least theoretically, and it tapers off in both directions. It feels hotter in July and August, usually, but a part of that is due to increased humidity.

Regardless of age and season, of most immediate importance is time of day. You should be especially careful about exposure during the 12 noon to 2 P.M. period, when the sun is most directly overhead and hottest. The farther you can get from that two-hour period, the more exposure you can take. Thus, you will tan more safely from 8 A.M. (or before) to about 10:30, and from 4 P.M. or so till dark. And never let a haze or fog, even when it masks the sun, trap you in a sense of security. The ultraviolet is coming through as usual. Remember that the ultraviolet is a "cool" ray, unfelt by the skin's sensory system, which is what makes it so sneaky.

The degree of immunity—or danger—that your natural skin tone presents can be rated on a scale in terms of percentage; light blonds and some redheads absorb 19 to 45 percent of the sunlight reaching them; medium-toned and darker skins, 35 percent, more or less; East Indians and

Indians (though shades vary greatly), about 22 percent; and some blacks (again the range is wide), about 16 percent. It will be noted that blacks can indeed get sunburned —and they do—and the possibility of incurring serious skin damage through extended overexposure also is a danger from which they are not free.

First Aid for Sunburn

We come now to the crunch—what to do if wisdom has taken a summer's day off and that night the skin erupts in a disturbing glow.

Only partial relief is immediately possible, and the means are really quite simple. If the burn covers a fairly large portion of the body, take a cool bath without soap; a shower is too forceful at the moment for the skin's exquisite sensitivity—and cool water, contrary to an age-old belief, soothes any kind of burn and does not encourage blistering. On the reddest, painful parts apply cool, wet compresses, preferably soaked in Burow's solution,* available at any chemist.

If the burn does not seem severe, cover it with a mild emollient cream; a medicated cream is best avoided because it contains an antiseptic that, while ordinarily helpful, may prove irritating in this situation.

If the burn is more than mild, use one of the sunburn creams that contain either of two anesthetics, benzocaine or nupercaine (see the label). In the event of blistering or unusual temperature, or both, it is only good judgment to see the doctor at once. He will inject—or prescribe taking by mouth—a corticosteroid or an antihistamine, which will afford the quickest, most complete relief possible. In any case, whether the burn is severe or mild, carefully avoid any further exposure to the sun until pain and redness are entirely gone.

---

* Aluminium Acetate Solution, B.P.C.

Suntanning and Sunscreening Aids

When you next challenge the sun you should be wearing —as you should have been in the first place—an ample coating of a "suntan" cream or oil which, as I have already noted, does nothing to cause tanning but does keep out most of the ultraviolet rays' sunburning portions. It is not an all-day filter and needs to be replenished every hour or so, depending on the sun's intensity. Give special attention to those parts of the skin that are thinnest, such as the eyelids. There are some parts of the body that tend to burn faster than others, and you have probably noticed that about the nose, forehead, and the area just under the eyes. So more frequent attention should be given to these skin sectors as well as to a few others that burn with special ease—lips, ears, kneecaps, and the foot's instep.

A most important fact to understand is that *no* sunscreening preparation will ensure complete immunity to sunburn. Dr. John M. Knox of Baylor University has pointed out that the preparations should be far more effective than they are. Consult your doctor, who will suggest the most effective sunscreening lotion. The commercial sunscreen is offered in one hundred or more brand names and most of them rely largely on the ingredient para-aminobenzoic acid (with para often denoted simply as p-). Two other common bases are menthyl anthranilate and homo-menthyl salicylate, but they appear to be less effective. A total sunblock, which eliminates the possibility of sunburn but also interferes sharply with tanning, usually contains benzophenone.

Warding Off Sunburn: Summary

These, then, are the general guidelines for avoiding your undoing by the sun:

- Approach the summer warily. Not more than thirty

minutes of sun the first day, with only small increases each day until tanned.

• Only "mad dogs and Englishmen go out in the midday sun," wrote Noel Coward, an Englishman. He did not say how it affected them, but they, I'm quite sure, suffer from it just as much as any other group does.

• Use a sunscreening product of proved effectiveness, renewing the coating as needed, and always after coming out of the water.

• Before going into the sun, take no drugs and use no cosmetics that may make your skin photosensitive.

• After each exposure use an emollient, moisturizing, or good face cream to offset the dryness the sun has caused.

• For painful or even uncomfortable sunburn, use a sunburn lotion that contains an anesthetic. For an unusually severe case, see your doctor.

• Should long overexposure bring on "liver spots"—the brownish blotches more accurately called sebhorreic keratodes—see your doctor or a dermatologist. This condition is strongly suspected of being precancerous and is best treated at once. Treatment has been very successful with fluorouracil (5-FU), applied externally each day for several weeks. If they do not wholly fade, the spots can be removed by electrodesiccation.

I am aware that I have filled this chapter with warnings, precautions, and other negative observations regarding the sun. I have referred entirely to *overexposure* of normal skins and even brief exposure of skins that react abnormally to the sun. Having taken exception to the cult of the heliophile—the sun-lover—it should not be assumed that I am a heliophobe.

I enjoy the sun, but knowing it for the enemy that it can be, I enjoy it on my own terms, not the sun's. Our relationship, one might say, is at arm's length.

But if the sun's ultraviolet rays can be avoided or rendered impotent—by methods I have related—sunbathing will contribute to your health by stimulating the circulation, thereby engendering a feeling of health, a sense of well-being. It is known to relieve acne and minor skin problems.

Lying in the sun will rest and relax you, providing some respite from the tensions that afflict us all. But the cautions still hold.

And, finally, it may soon be possible for even the most dedicated heliophile to eat his cake and have it, though some measure of moderation will still be needed.

Today there are pills that are believed to hasten the sun-tanning process and thus reduce the danger of sunburning. They contain *psoralen,* and in most areas require a prescription. It has been reported that a vitamin, pyridoxine, in doses of 1200 milligrams daily, will also be helpful. Dr. Edward Mandel has described the beneficial effect of this treatment in the *New York State Journal of Medicine.* Still another sunburn preventative that has been recommended is—would you believe it?—aspirin. Taking ten grains (two tablets) of aspirin one hour before sunning may also reduce the harmful effects of the sun and may produce a better tan. If the aspirin can be combined with an anti-histamine, the beneficial effects should be enhanced.

To protect photosensitive patients requires the use of a complete sun block such as Uval®, or Uvistal®, Solebar®, Spectraban®, or of Reflecta®, Ardena Covering Cream® or medicated Make-Up® with a sunscreen, to wear on sunny days.

9

Are You Aging? Ask Your Skin

Has the dread moment of truth now finally arrived? . . . when you ask yourself: "Is this it? Have I begun to show my age?"

The clue was not that extra bit of fatigue at the top of that familiar staircase. Nor that sudden, vague wish to stay close to the television set this Saturday night instead of going out.

It was something about your skin—the first mere trace of a few fine wrinkles at the corners of the eyes . . . a slight brittleness of the fingernails . . . the almost imperceptible veining of the hands (women say they look there first when secretly playing the guess-her-age game). And so, if you want to check your Visible Age Index (VAI —first mentioned by the author), consult your skin. It's the first to know.

Your Telltale Skin

If you are struck by a fear that what your skin tells you it also will tell others, you're right. Your skin will trumpet your plight to anyone who bothers to look.

Your first reaction is one of indignation and frustration. After all, you don't feel any older than you did, say, ten years ago. You've lost nothing essential of that young *feel-*

ing you've always had. Your waistline is still trim—well, nothing a couple of weeks of diet can't cure. Your physical vigor hasn't waned—anyhow, not *that* much. Your feeling about the opposite sex is undiminished—it's just that you have it under "better control" now. Certainly, your zest for life is still running in high gear—and no need to qualify that.

Those fine wrinkles, so slight that it took the magnifying mirror to show them up, are only among the first signs. The final, complete list of potential telltales can be frightening, though luckily not all of them are likely to happen to you. But slowly there is a deepening and spreading of these wrinkles; creases form where creases never were; there is a sagging of the skin, especially beneath the chin. While the uppermost layer of the facial surface coarsens, the total skin thickness diminishes. It loses its tone and elasticity, and when pinched or dented it springs back more slowly. Hair thins, of course, notably in the underarm and pubic areas, and in a man it becomes conspicuously sparser at the top, too.

At this time, hair growth otherwise takes opposite trends in the sexes. Male hair diminishes all over, particularly on the scalp, but women develop fuzz where there was none before—perhaps on the upper lip, where vertical ridges also deepen, and on other parts of the face. Pigmentation spots appear; so do moles and other brownish growths. With reduced secretion of body oils and perspiration, the skin dries. Its nourishment slows as circulation ebbs.

The Nature and Causes of Aging

What is "aging," that some show it at thirty and others not until after fifty?

The *what* of aging, the changes it brings, are well known. The *why* is still pretty much a mystery. But take heart. There are indeed reputable, eminent scientists who have found some persuasive clues and they hold that, under the right supervision, aging can be significantly delayed, even if it cannot be postponed indefinitely. Studies are being made, however, of new chemicals that some scientists believe may make it possible to clip years from one's appearance permanently.

Science is giving increasing attention not only to the aging process and the means of retarding it, but also to deferring its visible signs. Together with this increase in interest a single theory has, in the past decade, gained ever wider acceptance.

It is overexposure to the sun, more than any other single factor, that ages the skin before its time—and in most people. Increased tensions are an important secondary factor. While the causes of aging skin are more than one, however, the evidence indicting the sun is too significant to aquit it of a heavy burden of blame.

It would be unreasonable to reject other scientifically acceptable doctrines that have found answers within a broader context. Dr. Hans Selye of McGill University, Montreal, believes we age because we wear out unevenly, and that if we could learn to balance the use of our various parts in our earlier years, aging and death would come much later. Dr. Robert Wilson, a prominent New York gynecologist and author of the book *Forever Feminine,* firmly advocates the thesis that the taking of female hormones in a closely supervised program will permit a woman to skip menopause completely, and that she will be menstruating in her sixties (though the reproductive capacity will vanish at the usual age). This prolonged youthfulness, he says, will also be manifested by a "younger" skin, an absence of such menopausal symptoms as flushes, an avoidance of depression and tension, and a full restoration of abandoned sex patterns. My own clinical experience supports Dr. Wilson to the extent that some of my women patients who regularly take the estrogen-progestin (female

hormone) contraceptive pills have observed that this practice has been accompanied by a healthier-looking skin, re-
flecting a more radiant glow, with facial lines becoming less
evident. The hormones prescribed by Dr. Wilson have a
strong resemblance to the contraceptive pills; indeed, he
sometimes directs the use of the latter for antiaging pro-
grams.

With natural estrogen, Dr. Wilson suggests cyclic treatment seven days off and twenty-one days on every month.
No medication is given the rest of the month.

There can no longer be much question that the aging
symptoms are sharply accelerated by the slowing activity
of the sex glands as the years mount. The dwindling production of sex hormones in both men and women is a
major factor in the overall conspiracy to promote the evil
process of aging.

The estrogen maturation factor is used to determine
normal secretion of estrogen. Many people are worried
about the possibility of estrogen causing breast or genital
cancer. However, Dr. Harry Leis, Jr., Clinical Professor of
Surgery at New York Medical College, reported after
studies of the results of estrogen therapy in patients who
had been given this treatment from ten to fourteen years
that not one case of cancer developed among these people.
Dr. Robert Wilson reported on 304 women whom he had
treated with estrogen over a period of twenty-seven years.
Not a single case of cancer had appeared among them. So,
if you are taking estrogen, relax.

Another responsible medical scientist has pointed a
stern finger at diet as a major factor in aging. As people get
older and their energy needs subside, they eat less. Because
they then become thinner, they give less attention to "diet,"
which they have usually associated with weight control.
They tend to abandon a balanced diet. They may avoid the
wrong foods, but that is not enough. They simply do not
eat enough of the *right* foods. Dr. Benjamin Frank, a med-

ical researcher, writes that aging skin can be improved markedly by a diet high in ribonucleic acid along with high potency Vitamin B complex capsules and foods containing purine. The theory is credible and Dr. Frank has supported it by citing a number of cases in which this combination has shown dramatic results in reversing skin deterioration. The improvement he attributes to the effect of the RNA and Vitamin B complex on the fibrous tissues, collagen, and elastic fibrils under the skin. RNA is no faddish thing. This basic, protein-related substance has been called "the body's building blocks" and the essential "key to life." It is basic in every living cell; all cellular and molecular processes relate to it. The discovery of ribonucleic acid's influence was a massive step toward a more complete understanding of the processes of living—and aging.

But there remains more to be said about the effect of the sun—or its man-made substitute, the ultraviolet lamp—on the skin. The mention of old age might provoke an image of a senior citizen lazing in the sun, absorbing its health-giving rays and its unique regenerative benefits. Taken in very moderate doses, the sun does offer some muscular relaxation and provides a small amount of Vitamin D. In any larger dose, as we saw in the last chapter, the sun can become a merciless enemy, whatever your age, and there is abundant evidence that it is the frequent cause of skin cancer. The conclusion of Dr. Knox, whose investigations of the sun's effect on the skin were cited in the preceding chapter, is emphatic:

"The visible cutaneous [skin] changes usually interpreted as aging in skin are due largely, if not entirely, to sunlight."

Largely, perhaps. Entirely, probably not. At the same medical symposisum at which Dr. Knox made his valuable disclosures, another light was beamed on the problem of aging skin by Dr. Richard B. Stoughton of Western Reserve University Medical College, Cleveland. He granted that overexposure to sunlight was a likely factor in skin aging, but he made a convincing case for other causes too—hormonal reduction, tension, strain, and the cumulative effect of anxieties. He added some fascinating disclosures about means of retarding the entire aging process, which had been achieved with laboratory animals. Their life spans had been extended by diet at a near-starvation level, by keeping them in a constantly cool atmosphere, and by reducing their basal metabolism rate, which is the measure of the amount of energy expended when the subject is at complete rest. It was not suggested that these courses were now realistic for human application, but it seems not impossible that they will one day be.

Hope for Aging Skin: Dos and Don'ts

Meanwhile, there *is* hope for the aging skin, even the skin that seems well down the road to total ruin. The help of a skilled dermatologist can make a vast difference, but while you're thinking about seeing one, there are a number of vitally important things you can do—and *not* do—for yourself. Start with these recommendations:

Do *not,* except for very brief periods, expose hands or face to the sun's rays without protective sun hat and an effective sunscreening cream or lotion. The sun's "corrugation" of the skin is often irreversible. If sunburn occurs, treat it at once. A suntan may suggest health, but it isn't necessarily so. Gradual exposure to the sun's rays is best.

Do *not* assume that the only benefit of diet control is weight control. Correct diet means proper balance of *all* essential nutrients, and for seniorish citizens the emphasis must be on proteins, unsaturated fats, fruits, vegetables, trace minerals, and vitamins. A low starch intake is advisable. The controversy over organic foods versus nonorganic foods is not solvable at present.

In general, for all patients over fifty who have skin changes, I routinely suggest 25,000 units of Vitamin A per day, 500 milligrams of Vitamin C, and an all-purpose vita min and mineral capsule. These are the vitamins needed for production and maintenance of skin integrity in the aging. In older people, there is usually poor absorption and selection of foods and slowed metabolism, so supplement ing the diet with vitamins and minerals is desirable. Occasionally, a capsule containing betaine hydrochloride and/or intestinal enzymes may be desirable to help with the digestion of foods. I suggest also 800 units of Vitamin E (alphatocopherol). I have been clinically treating patients with a new moisturizing cream containing the related sup plements alantoin polygalacturonic acid and alantoin ribonucleic acid in an acid mantle base. The results look promising.

The generally safe cosmetics sold these days not only pleasantly conceal the unkind traces of the years but also can be of strong benefit to the skin, especially the moistur izing creams that temporarily ameliorate dryness.

Do *not* ride in a top-down convertible. If the sun doesn't smite the flesh the wind will. Excessive basking in the sun on a boat without proper protection may be devastating.

Do *not* force smiling or frowning. They're allies of wrinkling. Of course, a smile prompted by genuine pleas ure or humor is a natural act.

To this list of *do nots*, it might be added that there is more bad news for smokers. Dr. Harry W. Darnell, a California internist, after examining the photographs of 1,104 persons with crow's-feet, found that there was an association between cigarette smoking and wrinkles. The correlation was even greater when smoking was associated with outdoor exposure.

Dr. Darnell, who has been studying the relationship be tween smoking and wrinkles since 1957, admits that there is no single, specific cause for wrinkles. His article, which appeared in *Annals of Internal Medicine,* states: "The association between cigarette smoking and wrinkling can be readily confirmed by the interested, even though untrained observer, at any public gathering where the faces and smoking habits of individuals can be compared. In such a setting almost all strikingly wrinkled, relatively young persons are seen to be active smokers."

The benzopyrene in cigarette smoke is the noxious element responsible for this effect.

On the other hand, *do* try these suggestions out:

Follow most carefully the directions for avoiding excessive exposure to the sun and for minimizing the sun's harmful effects upon your skin given in the preceding chapter.

Keep the skin clean but without excessive washing—and never wash with very hot water. Use soap sparingly. Soap is drying, akaline, and the detergent types are even more so. Avoid excessive washing with harsh detergents. Be most frugal with soap and water in cold weather. The superfatted and transparent soaps are less drying. The use of cleansing cream is advisable; this product contains a moisturizer and a cleaning agent.

Establish a daily beauty routine along the lines suggested below. It's a habit you'll find relaxing and pleasurable—and will surely pay off in a younger, healthier appearance.

Keep nails of fingers and toes trimmed closely to discourage injury and splitting that years encourage. The intake of gelatin, organic calcium, and Vitamin B complex may help.

Squinting causes wrinkles. If you're inclined to squint, see an oculist who can abolish your habit by prescribing proper glasses—and be sure the frames fit comfortably.

Keep your living quarters well humidified, especially during the winter heating season.

Unless physical limitations counsel otherwise, continue actively the forms of daily exercise that bring order to your

life and fresh blood to the arterial vessels—pleasant house-
work, calisthenics, jogging, walking, and perhaps some en-
joyable athletic sport such as tennis or golf. Joining a well-
regulated, supervised gym is advisable.

Finally, maintain a sensible attitude about the aging
process. It's going to appear eventually, but play the game
of trying to hold it off—or slow it down—as long as possible.
Many people find the game is fun, and they feel hopeful
about it. Get grim about it and you're a sure loser. A positive program is better than a negative attitude.

A Cosmetic Regimen for the Middle and Later Years

What about the cosmetic routine? It is just a daily application of fine cosmetics to maintain skin health. Proper
cosmetics maintain the suppleness of the skin. Observe the
following regimen:

1. Keep the skin clean—reasonably clean is enough.
2. Cleanse with mild, superfatted, or clear soap—nondetergent—or with cleansing cream or lotion; use mildly
warm water and face cloth, and then cold.
3. If your skin is dry, as it may be, lubricate it with
natural vegetable oils like seasame, olive, peanut, apricot
kernel, safflower, or avocado oil. The chemist has them,
but so does the supermarket.
4. By day, use moisturizing cream before applying
makeup.
5. At night, remove the makeup with soap, cleansing
cream, or mineral oil (Albolene). Then apply moisturizing
and emollient creams. Leave them on all night, and in most
cases they will be absorbed.
6. For impurities arising on the skin due to air pollution, wash well with a good antiseptic soap. If a home sauna
device is available, use it cautiously with reference to the

affected area; if not, ordinary steaming will help. In any case, dry thoroughly and apply a thin coat of moisturizing cream.

7. It is desirable occasionally to use an astringent, such as witch hazel or diluted alcohol, to tone the skin and temporarily reduce the pores.

8. When the facial skin is exposed to the sun during the working day, use a foundation lotion or cream which contains a sunblocking agent.

Wrinkles and Lines

There is no known cosmetic or therapeutic preparation which will reduce wrinkles rapidly. Various remedies for facial lines have been recommended in popular publications and may be of help in some cases. Among them are massaging of the areas involved, and facial isometric exercises. (Exercises that exert a force against an opposing force are called isometric.) In these exercises the skin and tissues of the throat and forehead are drawn upward by action of the facial muscles, at the same time massaging gently with the fingers. Five minutes of this in the morning and five minutes at night may help in reducing minor lines. However, since it is deficiencies in the normal elasticity of the tissues, and in their collagen that cause lines and wrinkles, these remedies cannot be of much use in controlling the larger ones.

Recently a prominent television makeup man has developed an isometric "beauty band" which he claims lifts and smooths sagging facial skin, also helping to firm and strengthen muscles and tissues. He states that when worn during the day the band takes up the slack contours of the face and gives it a smooth and vibrant look. I have not yet, however, had an opportunity to observe patients who have worn this device.

The use of an absorbing, softening cream, applied to the

face with an upward and outward motion for five to ten minutes at night, may help in reducing some of the facial lines.

A number of years ago several cosmetics containing albumen were introduced with a great deal of fanfare for temporarily reducing facial wrinkles. In the United States the FDA ordered these preparations removed from the market because of their makers' unsubstantiated claims. However, the application of *fresh* egg white will contract the skin and will temporarily improve disfiguring lines. The egg white should be placed in a clean dish and applied with a wooden, cotton-tipped applicator, in an outward direction.

Life History

Quite recently, a widow came to the office for help. She was about sixty-five years of age and when she had lost her husband some ten years earlier she had moved to Florida. She got a position as a saleswoman in a fashionable dress shop and was quite happy. Her off hours she spent in the sun to make up for a lifetime of sunless living in New York.

For her the sun was too much, too late. Her skin wrinkled badly and "age spots" became profuse. Her condition was unsightly enough for patrons of the store to ask the owner that they be served by someone else. Indeed, that reaction became so general that her usefulness to the shop came to an end—and so did her job.

Her married son in New York suggested that she come back and live with him, and she did. At that time he was a patient of mine, under treatment for a resistant acne, and he was responding well to therapy. He brought his mother to the office because she was depressed, grieving over the loss of her job and, more recently, of many of her friends.

A chemosurgical "skin peeling" was performed and the results were evident in three weeks. The facial lines became less apparent, the skin smoother, and the "old age" spots lost much of their conspicuous pigmentation.

She thereafter had to stay out of the sun or be diligent in the use of a sunscreening lotion. She was counseled on the use of cosmetics, with emphasis on moisturizers. The diet laid out for her included supplements of Vitamin A, B complex, C and E with mineral supplements. It all leaned toward foods high in proteins and purine, which is contained in fish and meat.

In a matter of a few more months, this woman's skin appeared to have shed many years. Her outlook and total personality changed remarkably for the better, and, she reported, her social life was becoming more active. Indeed, the last time I saw her she said something about getting married again, and I was led to believe the prospect was a likely one. What hope there was for her skin, she had plainly realized.

Hormonal Creams and the Aging Skin

It would be a serious omission not to mention here the rising use of "hormonal" creams, merely because the subject is highly controversial. As usually manufactured, these creams contain about 10,000 units of synthetic estrogen per ounce, while some add a small quantity of another female hormone, progesterone.

A consensus of the medical profession would now probably produce a sharp no-confidence vote in the hormonal creams, about the same as "royal jelly" would get. On the other hand, one group of well-known dermatologists has stated that the use of steroid creams by patients has reduced lines and improved the appearance of the skin. Writing in a scientific journal,* Drs. T. H. Sternberg, P. LeVan, and E. T. Wright report their clinical evaluation of one of

* *Current Therapeutic Research*, Vol. III, No. 11 (November, 1961), pp. 469–471.

these steroid creams containing pregnenolone. They assert that there have been strikingly beneficial results, and support these findings with controlled studies. The changes were dramatic indeed.

If, therefore, you feel inclined to use a steroid cream, try it for perhaps a month or two, then watch for favorable results. Even if you see them, suspend use for two or three months, then resume. But if there's no improvement, forget it.

Surgical and Chemical Treatments for Senior Skin

Now let us suppose you're a Johnny-come-lately to the awareness of what can be done for the senior skin. It's become wrinkled, ridged, pigmented, moled, and rough. Dr. Wilson's prescribed female hormones may help—some. Dr. Frank's diet rich in ribonucleic acid and proteins should be quickly and permanently adopted—but your face still won't resemble a baby's.

In frustration, you ask, "Does it have to be this way always?"

No, it doesn't. There are the surgical and chemical remedies available to skilled and conscientious surgeons and dermatologists. If their approaches are not really for you, they will say so. If you come asking for a new and permanently regenerated face, they will turn you away, though gently. Their techniques can do much for your appearances—for two years, five years, ten years. Then, if the indications are right, the procedures *may* perhaps be repeated. Meanwhile, for you, time is not standing still. You *are* getting that much older. The clock can be turned back only so far.

A complete physical examination by a competent physician and dermatologist, and practical therapy, can be the first step toward renewed good health and an attractive skin. Perhaps the dermatologist may consider a "mechanical" treatment advisable. All these approaches are more or less radical, but results may be beneficial. Let's look at them more closely:

Plastic surgery: Commonly, the sagging skin is stretched, the overhangs are surgically removed, and edges are sutured together with remarkable skill and invisibility. How long the new, sag-free skin lasts depends on the depth of the surgery and the skill of the surgeon. Not all people or conditions are treatable. This procedure can be used for a face and eye lift.

In the "mini-lift," a small area of excessive, relaxed skin is removed from the back of the ear to produce a firmer appearance of the chin, cheeks, and cheekbone ridges. The effect lasts for only a short time.

Silicone injections: This technique is still experimental. Some plastic surgeons and dermatologists report good results, but others have warned of tissue damage. Silicone, a liquid, nonreactive chemical, is injected between the wrinkled skin and the underlying tissue. A resultant mild swelling tightens the skin, smoothing the wrinkles. Paraffin was formerly used in this way, but some injurious consequences caused it to be abandoned. Serious reactions to silicone breast implants have been reported.

Chemosurgery: This procedure is known as "skin peeling" or "modified chemoexfoliation." Used for reducing quite fine wrinkles and growths, it achieves some results with a caustic chemical. The skin is thoroughly cleaned and a paste containing resorcin, salicylic acid, or trichloroacetic acid plus phenol (carbolic acid) in some cases is applied to the involved area. Then, at a precise moment, the paste is removed and the acid chemical neutralized. Several days later, the skin peels away, removing superficial lines. The technique also helps stubborn pigmented patches. The Committee on Cosmetics of The American Medical Association has stated that chemosurgery is safe in the hands of a qualified skin specialist. The peeling removes the outer layer of skin and causes a swelling of the under layers, giving the impression of a smoother skin with fewer lines.

Dr. Perry A. Sperber of Daytona, Florida, has described the use of chemosurgery in his book *The Treatment of the Aging Skin and Dermal Defects*. He suggests that the results of peeling are temporary and have only moderate effect on deep lines.

It is important to bear in mind that this "peeling" process is safe only in the hands of a trained dermatologist who has first determined its suitability for his specific patient. The aftereffects are not very uncomfortable and the procedure may be repeated in a year or so. Because the chemicals are easily available, unqualified persons may offer such treatment. So think twice before turning your skin over to a beautician for a task only a specially trained doctor can handle.

Dermabrasion is sometimes referred as "skin planing." It is more painful and longer-lasting than chemosurgery, but its results may not be permanent either. It takes the utmost skill and practice for a dermatologist to use this technique successfully. The skin to be treated is cleaned, made aseptic, chilled, and anesthetized. Then a motor-driven, fine-wire brush is touched lightly to the treatment area with a motion that literally planes away acne pits and scarring. Healing takes a few weeks, and all traces of the planing have usually vanished in from six to eight weeks, seldom more. The first part of that period can be rather uncomfortable, but the new, smoother skin that results from the treatment makes it all worthwhile.

Which of these types of treatment the patient should undergo depends upon the degree of his or her motivations and upon the judgment of an experienced doctor as to which is most suitable in the circumstances.

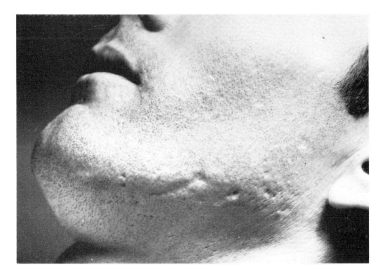

The smoothing effects of dermabrasion, or "skin
planing" by a skilled professional, are shown in
these photographs showing pitted skin (*above*)
and the same area after treatment (*below*).

(MARTIN HAGGERT PHOTOS)

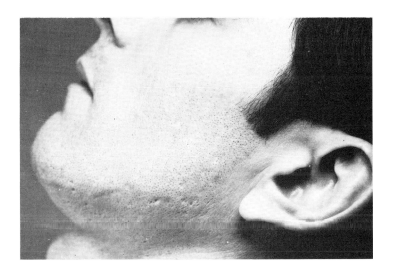

Stick to Sensible Measures

Many self-styled "spas" have appeared in the West Indies and other foreign countries, where cellular therapy and fertilized eggs were given to rejuvenate the tired and those seeking the Fountain of Youth. Their value, like that of the Niehans Therapy, has never been established. Basic good dieting, vitamins, hormones, a constructive outlook, and proper exercise will do more for the body and skin than all of these unproved, overtouted, and scientifically unrecognized treatments.

Often, the patient's problem is more psychological than physical. Ordinary, regular, day-to-day care of the skin as described in this chapter is the most practical and beneficial course.

Getting older—and showing it—is not easy for anyone to endure. Science can help a great deal, but an equally useful solution is to be found in a philosophical adjustment to what is inevitable—and really quite tolerable. To grow old gracefully is a satisfying achievement.

10

Pigmentation: Too Much and Too Little

In a world conscious of beautiful skin, the presence of excessive blotches and pigmentation on it can throw the unhappy bearer into a panic. These blotches may result from various causes, such as excessive sunburn or the internal use of pills which cause pigmentation when the skin is exposed to the sun. The pigmentation and photosensitivity go hand in hand.

Pigment-producing cells called melonocytes manufacture melanin, tiny dark particles that reside in the basal cell layer of the epidermis and are therefore not very far from the surface. The density of your melanin supply determines the shade of your complexion. At the two extremes, the blond skin contains the least of these pigment particles, the black skin the most.

It will not surprise you to learn that an individual's degree of pigmentation is entirely a matter of heredity, part of the genetic color scheme that affects the color of eyes and hair as well.

Between the blond and black skins come the colorings of such ethnic groupings as Italians, Greeks, and Spaniards (again with wide variations, depending upon racial mixtures); also somewhere in the middle ranges are the Asians —including but not limited to the Chinese and Japanese,

American Indians and Eskimos (both probably of Asiatic origin), peoples of the South Pacific, and virtually all other races not sharply identified as "white."

The anomaly is the albino, born with virtually no pigment in skin, eyes, and hair. If the eyes appear pinkish it is because the outer surface is so transparent, due to the lack of other color, that the blood in the subsurface vessels can be seen.

Because darker skin serves as better protection against the sun, we find blonds usually most sensitive to the ultraviolet rays, as we saw in Chapter 8. They burn rapidly without protection of shade, either the fixed kind of shade offered by tree or awning or the portable shade of the umbrella or wide-brimmed hat; if they risk the sun, between it and the skin there must be the ever-replenished barrier of sunblock or sunscreen lotion. On the other hand, the sunburning of a black skin, because it contains so much protective melanin, is rare, though not unknown. In the matter of terminology, excessive melanin production is called *hyperpigmentation;* when it is inadequate it's *hypopigmentation.*

Hyperpigmentation and Hypopigmentation

Chloasma: Another example of pigmentation gone out of control is chloasma or "liver spots" (see page 174). This abnormality causes the brownish, irregular pigment patches that may appear on the cheeks of pregnant women. After delivery, the patches most often turn lighter in color, and frequently they disappear. That is the hope, anyway.

If she chooses to avoid pregnancy by a regular routine of using contraceptive pills, a woman may also be inviting similar tannish pigment spots. That occurs in about 20 percent of the Pill's users and is actually a photosensitivity reaction—an irregular increase in melanin due to a biochemical action of the sun on the Pill's essential hormone, progesterone. During pregnancy, the body increases the progesterone supply; taking the Pill does about the same.

A similar erratic pigmentation is caused by the sun through photosensitization of skin areas that have been exposed to perfume containing oil of bergamot, as described in Chapter 6.

In dealing with problems of this kind, the most obvious way to diminish and to arrest hyperpigmentation is of course to stop the use of the Pill, perfume, or scented product. This act of self-denial will usually be necessary only in the summer months when the sun's ultraviolet rays are significant.

For the external counterattack, excessive pigmentation in patches may be further reduced by a bleaching cream containing hydroquinone. The cream, applied two or three times a day, will probably lighten the dark areas although they also may disappear entirely in a few months with patient effort.

Vitiligo: The reverse of chloasma is also a serious cosmetic problem. It arises with the irregular *reduction* of the melanin supply and causes unsightly white patches, lighter than the normal pigmentation of the involved skin. While sometimes loosely called "freckles in reverse," it is actually *vitiligo* (pronounced vittle-EYE-go). The patches appear on cheeks, hairline, fingers, neck, backs of hands, eyes, nose, nipples, navel, and genitals, though not necessarily on all. They are often observed in the normally darker-pigmented ethnic groups. Of course, "observed" may be misleading. It is likely that the light vitiligo spots are merely more conspicuous on darker skin. Luckily, only about 2 percent of the population is affected.

Except for the fact that about 40 percent of vitiligo patients report a hereditary factor, the cause is otherwise unknown. A few experimental approaches to treatment have been made, largely with little effect. Because the spots have little or no pigment, no amount of sun exposure will darken them; indeed, a suntan only makes the spots' contrast more visible.

However, the most promising treatment has been reported by an Egyptian physician, Dr. Abdul Mofty, of the University of Cairo. For patients with vitiliginous patches he instituted the use of psoralen compounds, both internally and externally, and recorded an effective return of normal pigmentation in from 30 to 60 percent of his cases.

In practice, I have found that the long-sustained use of these new chemicals, the psoralens, has been helpful in the normalization of pigmentation, although only in a small group of patients who were treated.

From time to time, one hears a suspicion voiced that vitiligo must be a spotty variety of albinism. This is not true; there is no relationship whatever. Vitiligo does not, for example, affect eye color as albinism does.

If the light, hypopigmented areas are on the face and prove embarrassing, they can be readily concealed with a masking cream or foundation lotion.

When any abnormality of skin pigmentation appears, it makes sense to consult a physician at once for a proper diagnosis and whatever treatment is available in the case.

Freckles: In children, freckles are considered "cute." When they carry over into adulthood, they may still have appeal but it is now more limited. Across the bridge of the nose, a few well-spaced freckles can be carried off very well by a pert-looking girl; a fully freckled face is generally considered a cosmetic misfortune, to say the least. Of course, that resistance is not universal—some of us are freckle-fanciers who enjoy them even in abundance.

Besides, at this juncture in our popular culture, some women who have been denied natural freckles acquire a few with judicious touches of an eyebrow pencil.

The *how* of freckles is well enough known but, again, the

why is not. They are simply brownish or reddish pigmentation spots darker than the surrounding skin. Babies aren't
born freckled—only with the susceptibility. They are first
brought out by exposure to the sun—"developed" rather
like a photographic print. It usually happens in the first
three years of infancy, accompanied by an overall suntan.
But when the tan fades, the spots refuse to go along with it
and little is known about discouraging them. Thus, while
freckles arrive by an abnormal process we know about, it
is this refusal to vanish that is mysterious and more vexing.

If you have freckles and the word somehow offends you,
take some comfort in knowing that your disorder of pigmentation is known as *ephilides.*

True, there are some moderate frecklers lucky enough to
have the chameleon ability to shuck them off as summer
wanes. For others, the lightness or darkness of the spots
varies little over the seasons, though their visibility changes.
In winter, when the skin has resumed its usual lightness,
the darker freckles stand out more. But a summer's suntan,
if dark, will make them paler than surrounding skin.

While freckling usually originates in infancy, as noted,
it may appear for the first time in adolescence or adulthood,
but these are the cases more likely to be a seasonal phe-
nomenon; at summer's end, the freckles may vanish, or
decide to stay.

Everyone has noted that redheads, though lacking an
exclusive franchise, are most prone to freckling. It probably
has something to do with the bizarre pigmentation that
made them redheads in the first place.

For the freckle-prone, the best course must be very clear—
avoid overexposure to the sun. Once the damage is done,
there is no sure "cure." The hydroquinone cream used for
chloasma may help, but only by temporary bleaching.
There is nothing that will penetrate the skin deeply
enough to affect the melanocytes that control the pigmentation pattern.

For many generations, home-remedy techniques have been tried; none has been of avail and some can be disastrous to the skin. An old one is undiluted lemon juice, but it's more useful in lemonade on a warm day. Mild chemosurgery can individually peel off the freckles. Occasionally application of hydroquinone cream will help.

If you are freckle-prone and must go out in the sun, cover up all exposed areas with a basecoat of a good sunscreening cream or lotion to block the freckle-forming ultraviolet rays. When the ointment dries, apply a cover-up makeup in a shade blending with your normal color. If you're going swimming or are likely to perspire a good deal, the makeup should be of a waterproof type that needs soap for removal. The beauty experts say that this waterproof top coat, when it sets, should be buffed with a soft, dry cloth—such as Turkish toweling—for a natural skin appearance.

11

Allergies

There must be more agreeable ways to prove it, but the existence of allergies—for no clear reason afflicting some and leaving others totally immune—offers firm evidence that we are indeed a world of differents. If allergy somehow separated the men from the boys, the women from the girls, it would have an inherent logic. But it makes no distinctions, falling alike on the just and the unjust.

Some 30 percent of us are allergy-prone to some degree, enough to have brought the word "allergy" into broad currency and, inevitably, loose definition. We say "allergy" when we mean "allergic reaction" or "allergen," which is the central substance involved in a reaction. We say we are allergic to someone we don't like, although we are often allergic to things we love. (People allergic to strawberries would never know it if they didn't eat them.)

Almost every form of matter known to humans—animal, vegetable, mineral . . . liquid, solid, gas—can produce an allergic reaction in someone, somewhere. Quite suddenly, for no reason immediately apparent, the skin will raise a rash—or blisters or swelling, usually with itching. Or the sinuses begin to act up. Or the eyes water. Or there is sneezing or coughing. In acute cases, breathing may become very difficult, perhaps even impossible; some insect bite reactions prove fatal.

Fortunately, most reactions are mild and transient; even before we begin to take them seriously they are gone. The eyes may tear a bit, a mild itch is casually scratched, a runny nose routinely wiped, and that's about it. But for some people an allergy can mean a life of tyranny, limitation, and unending discomfort.

Allergy may be broadly described as *hypersensitivity*. For reasons the body knows best but is not telling us, it rebels against something that is touched, swallowed, inhaled, or injected. Does it rebel against your nail polish? Not really. It's resenting something *in* the polish, and that specific something is the *allergen*. If you switch to some hypoallergenic polish, containing none of the most likely of the known allergens, your skin will probably soon be entirely in the clear.

Actually, we know a good deal about allergy except, alas, Fact No. 1—the secret of why one human system will hotly dispute the presence of some substance while another will ignore it.

Well known, however, is what happens when an allergen invades. The reaction doesn't usually happen at once, and seldom with the first invasion. But at some time—with perhaps the fourth invasion or the fortieth or the hundredth—the body's defenses lose control over the persistent intrusions. They engage the allergen, determined to neutralize its violence. In the ensuing conflict, a chemical known as histamine is released into the system, causing a biochemical reaction. It is this part of the process that brings on the rash, the wheezing, the tears, or the other annoying symptoms.

The antibodies sometimes win, though it's a victory of philosophical realism. They don't eject the allergen; they merely enable the body to live with it. They seek to confer future immunity.

If they fail and the reactions persist, the afflicted victim must either get adjusted to bearing that cross indefinitely, or more wisely, see a doctor. The family physician or a dermatologist (or allergist) may succeed where the antibodies failed. He may proceed with a course of desensitization, but before that he must identify the allergen, which can be very difficult.

As I remarked earlier, identification is a form of detective work, but it is done the way good detectives operate— methodically, painstakingly . . . the hard way—by a process of elimination. The doctor uses patch or scratch tests. Tiny quantities of known, common allergens—scores of them—are mixed in specific groupings and a bit of each is scratched into the skin, usually on the arm, in a regular pattern. The scratches are covered and about twenty-four hours later are exposed for inspection. If one scratch shows marked redness or a welt, the reaction is called positive and the doctor knows he has picked up a live trail, and all the other test allergens have been exonerated. The mixture that caused the positive reaction is next broken down into its component allergen samples and they are scratched into the skin individually. The one (perhaps two, three, or more) that now shows a positive reaction is the villain.

The desensitization stage follows. Again, small quantities of the offending allergen (s) are used, but this time they are injected just under the skin. With each visit, the dose is increased and, in time, the system learns to tolerate them very well. Sometimes the same goal can be achieved by a do-it-yourself approach, provided some food is the offender and you have been able to identify it. Simply eat small quantities of that food until you build up a tolerance for it. But a scientific course of desensitization is much quicker— and surer. Desensitization is not, however, always successful.

Allergens and Their Friends

The allergens, then, come in four major forms:

1. *Inhalants*—breathed in
2. *Ingestants*—swallowed
3. *Contactants*—touched
4. *Injectants*—something penetrating the skin.

When the body has finally decided to act against a persistent intruder—the allergen—the situation has reached the "critical threshold," and the action begins. The allergen hasn't done it alone, though. The threshold stage arrives only if other conditions also are present—perhaps a respiratory infection, overexercise, a disorder of the sinuses or ears, or a low level of gamma globulin that indicates inadequate production of the essential antibodies.

A change in humidity—or an emotional upset—might be all the allergen needs. Hives in particular are often provoked emotionally, and an attack may quickly retreat or it may stay around a long time. In some cases, only psychotherapy helps.

There is believed to be a heredity factor involved in allergy, though not always. A parent who is allergic, say, to feathers does not necessarily pass that sensitivity on; the child may be affected only by eggs or oysters. Two sisters may have wholly different allergies, or one may have none at all. The theory is that the factor inherited is a defect in the cell chemistry. It also has been observed by dermatologists that a patient with a specific allergy may often have a tendency to other allergies.

The Most Troublesome Allergens

Most allergies are provoked by dust, chemicals, polluted air, perfumes, foods, and drugs, representing the four provocative groups of substances—breathed in, swallowed, touched, and injected.

Conspicuous among those *inhaled* are house dust, gasoline fumes, hairs or dust from such animals as horses or cats, numerous plant pollens and pillow feathers, as well as tobacco smoke. Most of these may touch off an attack of asthma or hay fever in those who are sensitive, but reactions may show up on the skin as well.

The *ingestants* (swallowed) can cause skin reactions too, but more commonly they trigger nausea or diarrhea. The list of possible allergy-spurring foods is endless, but most frequently they are fish, shellfish, strawberries, milk products, eggs, citrus fruits, pork, soybeans, spices, nuts, and chocolate.

The *injectants* may be regarded as a subgroup of the ingestants because they also enter the body, though without being swallowed. They penetrate it through the physician's hypodermic syringe or the sting of an insect, which can be extremely dangerous. The one most often causing a reaction (perhaps because it is the one most often injected) is penicillin. If you have in the past reacted badly to it, tell your doctor when he has occasion to use it. Fortunately, he has other, equally effective antibiotics. The sulfa drugs, tetracycline, declamycin, aureomycin and other antibiotics may possibly run head-on into some sensitivities, but few people react adversely to all of them.

After all, a significant number of people cannot tolerate even aspirin and sensitivity is frequent to barbiturates sometimes found in sleeping pills. Also to be watched for reactions are bromides, iodides, and the contraceptive pill.

Among the *contactants,* those creating the most problems are a very broad range of chemicals and cosmetics. The most annoying contactant, however, is poison ivy, followed by poison oak and poison sumac. However, gardeners often find they must stay clear of contact with primulas, tulip bulbs, geraniums, gladioli, and chrysanthemums.

In a practical sense, the most serious allergies are those afflicting people exposed to them in their trades or professions. If desensitization does not work, means can often be found to help them by-pass exposure; but if that is not possible they must look for other forms of livelihood even though that can mean a wrecked career and a permanently reduced standard of living. It is significant, though, that most of these people experience a first reaction only after many thousands of exposures.

That was true of the dentist I treated for severe, painful rashes of both hands. They were cracked, red, and rough. Tracing his problem to the source was a complex task, but at last we struck it. For performing extractions and other painful procedures, the anesthetic of his choice was xylocaine. But whatever pain xylocaine was sparing his patients was being, in a sense, absorbed by his agonized hands. The solution was simple enough: he changed to another anesthetic and, for as long as it took his hands to get the message, he used some protective creams I prescribed.

The vocation that, in my experience, poses most problems of occupational allergy—also described as contact eczematous dermatitis—is that of operators in beauty salons. And small wonder. For hours each day their hands are assailed by a bewildering variety of cosmetic products containing rich mines of potential allergens—in hair dyes, permanent waving and hair-straightening solutions, nail polish, shampoos, soaps, setting lotions, assorted sprays, lanolin, chemical preservatives, emulsifiers, and many other products containing perfumes.

The beauty shop employee with any such sensitivity is in deep trouble since it is impossible to wear protective gloves for all jobs; even protective creams are sometimes impractical. The only alternative seems to be a change in vocations.

There are many industries that show a high incidence of occupational dermatitis because of the products they use. Those posing most such problems, according to an extensive government study, manufacture synthetic resins, chemicals, and dyes. The classes of materials creating the most employee skin problems are petroleum products, greases, and alkalis (cement included). In recent years, industries have adopted practices and measures to avoid such trouble, but total eradication seems impossible because human sensitivities vary so much. I have found that an affected worker can usually remain on the job in such a hostile environment by shielding exposed skin with a silicone cream called Rosalex, which provides an invisible barrier.

Considering the hazards of such workers within the context of the total population, they probably are not very significant statistically. But the world's most common occupation offers singular exposure to contact dermatitis—that of the housewife. Appendix I in this book gives an awesome, but only partial, inventory of the aggressors that each day emerge from her kitchen closets to assault her skin. Just a few are her detergents, soaps, polishes, insecticide, oven cleaner, chlorinated soap, scouring powder, ammonia, laundry bleach, and wax remover. She must learn by alertness which are most abusive and either avoid or replace them. Whether or not that is possible, she should wear rubber gloves and use protective creams abundantly.

Dog owners have always been exposed to dog hairs and dust, making many of them susceptible. Often, a romp through a poison ivy patch has left some of the evil plant oil on the coat of the dog, who has returned home to an owner who pets him, with an unhappy outcome. A new hazard now appears in the form of the antiflea collar that has become popular. Drs. P. C. Cronce and H. S. Alden of the Emory University School of Medicine, Atlanta, Georgia, have reported some cases of contact dermatitis traced to the insecticide the collar contains. It is soluble in water and when the dog becomes wet the insecticide spreads over his coat; some people are highly sensitive to it.

Photoallergy, which I have already described on pages

113–114, is an allergy caused by direct sunshine. Most of us can avoid the penalties of excessive sun just by being sensible. Some people, however, are inherently photosensitive, which means uniquely and most disagreeably affected by even small doses of sunlight. For them, prevention demands heroic measures, even to the extreme of living in shaded rooms by day and going outdoors only after sunset lest they contract a sunburn—in effect, a poisoning—far more villainous than anything that the rest of us ever experience.

Inevitably, new products appear in the marketplace and become used for the purpose of improving, somehow, the human condition. One of the prices we pay for such improvement is the broadening of the range of adverse human reactions.

Among the more recent objects of suspicion are the deodorant soaps, which generally have proved useful to many although even that value is being minimized. These soaps have relied heavily upon an antiseptic ingredient to control the bacteria that cause body odors. Initially, the antibacterial agent was hexachlorophene, which is indeed very effective. But investigators came up with a finding that experiments with a *limited* number of rats—given exposure to *massive* doses of hexachlorophene over a two-year period, which does not seem to relate well to normal human use— have shown that about 25 percent of the rats developed brain damage; an additional number showed lesser symptoms of that order.

While a controversy raged, many manufacturers using hexachlorophene in deodorant soaps switched to another antiseptic, TBS (tribromsalicylanilide), although some had always been using it instead of hexachlorophene. Almost at once, dermatologists in different parts of the country reported that TBS was a photosensitizer causing skin eruptions. Their charges covered not only deodorant soaps but also after-shave lotions using TBS. These products made some patients so photosensitive, they said, that they reacted even to sunlight filtering through a window or to the light from a fluorescent lamp.

The makers of the soaps and lotions protested that even if such a hazard did exist, too few people were affected to deprive the vast majority of the benefits of TBS. The dermatologists conceded the number was small but, they said, since anyone who bathes regularly doesn't need a deodorant soap, anyway, why risk trouble?

What to Do About Allergy and Such

If any allergy or a related sensitivity should mark you as one of its own, it may be a small comfort to know that you don't really have a "skin disease" but only a reaction to something eaten, breathed in, or touched, or to some injections that your body's *protective system* finds hostile. It shows up on the skin only because that is where you can see it.

Your first countermeasure must be the calm question: "In the past seventy-two hours or less, what have I eaten, touched or breathed in that I don't ordinarily? Have I had an injection?" A new food or new cosmetic—or an old one in a new form? New bedding, a new cat, a new drug, a new fabric in stockings or underwear? New elastic somewhere?

That first question can be the critical one and, if stubbornly pursued, is the likeliest to produce the right answer. Run down all of the suspects suggested earlier in this chapter. If that yields nothing, keep trying. As each possibility pops into your mind, ask another question: "Have I ever heard of anyone being sensitive to that?"

From your list of suspicious characters, banish all contact with *only one* of them for about three days. If that changes nothing, do the same with the others, each in turn.

Should you find that the avoidance of one seems to turn the trick, form no firm conclusion without double-checking; that is, try again a small exposure to it—food, drug, inhalant, contactant. If the reaction returns, cast the guilty substance from your life.

But if this procedure doesn't work for you and a reaction persists, lose no more time in getting to your family doctor, to a dermatologist, or an allergist. He will probably begin the patch-test series and perhaps start desensitization in an effort to immunize you to whatever it is that ails you.

Because sensitivities can be extremely complex, desensitization is not always possible and avoidance of your allergen as a defensive measure is not always practical.

In extreme cases, where the condition proves to be intractable, it may become necessary to abandon a vocation where exposure to a specific allergen is unavoidable, or to move from a neighborhood where an allergic hazard is present without recourse.

In any case, at least temporary relief is possible. The doctor will prescribe an antihistamine or will inject a corticosteroid that will prove most helpful until his longer-range treatment takes effect.

Accenting the Cosmetics Allergy

Most allergic reactions, especially among city dwellers, are of the contact type. Narrowing them down to women, a large share of their adverse reactions, if not most of them, arise from cosmetics they cannot tolerate, or for which they develop an intolerance even after long use.

An easily checked chart—listing the various cosmetics by type, the possible allergens they contain, and the kind of symptoms that most often result—has been prepared by the Ar-Ex Products Company, a cosmetics producer, and has

been featured by the publication *Hairdo & Beauty*. I consider the chart to be comprehensive and useful. Your
need—and your instinct for what may be troubling you—
might sometime lead you to consult it. It is given in Appendix I.

12

Dermatitis Urbis, or City Skin

The farmer is bronzed to a glow of health by the sun's life-giving ultraviolet rays that penetrate the pure, clean, unpolluted air in which he lives all day. So is the sailor. Those pure, life-giving ultraviolet rays that bronze them can also give them skin cancer, or, with some luck, only a pre-cancerous skin condition. These growths are known as "solar" keratodes, which appear on the sun-exposed surfaces of the face and are red, warty, and irregular in appearance.

Both sailor and farmer are outdoorsmen. Most of us are not. We live and/or work in cities. In America city dwellers were a minority as recently as the 1960s when the urban/rural balance in the population shifted to the urban. Small farmers were selling out to larger ones and moving their families to the big towns.

The relocated farm families traded their clean air and relatively pure water for the environmental conditions we urbanites somehow endure, and they became exposed to our hazards. There is a body of scientific opinion—still lacking either solid support or final disproof—that holds that the lifelong city dweller somehow develops a good measure of tolerance for the brutal urban environment.

Considering that we do stay alive in it, the theory may be sound.

However, it seems to apply largely to respiratory diseases. In at least one other respect—the skin—we are by no means unscathed. Indeed, I have for several years been treating a skin ailment mentioned in none of the medical literature. In time I came to identify this unique disorder—in fact, a combination of disorders—as being peculiar to city dwellers. These findings were later confirmed by an English physician.

For its quick identification, I needed a name for it. Logic and realism dictated the generic term *dermatitis urbis*, which in English comes down to "City Skin." Why does it happen?

Even city folk are scarcely aware of all their atmospheric assailants, but their magnitude is suggested by a brief inventory.

To begin with, Dr. Morris Jacobs of the Columbia University School of Public Health, a specialist in air pollution, says that the New Yorker's chief environmental enemy is the fumes from the fuel burned in the city—fuel oil and bituminous coal. Despite a relatively new municipal law restricting the sulfur content of fuel oil, its smoke fogs the city with sulfur dioxide. And few other cities have any such restriction.

The exhausts of cars moving slowly through the jammed streets contribute acrolein, an organic compound; it comes also from building incinerators as they burn fats and send other cremated, powdered garbage to mix with the air we breathe and literally touch.

Car exhausts offer also such other nonboons as carbon monoxide, benzoprene, tars, nitrogen oxides, and ethyl lead. And the ozone that gets into the atmosphere from photochemical reactions may be enough to cause emphysema or other broncho-pulmonary disorders.

That catalogue should be depressing enough, but there

are also soot and dust from many sources other than fuel, and they help bacteria to prosper; from the burned coal comes fly ash too, and there are dog droppings and varying amounts of radioactivity.

If you live in a city other than seriously polluted New York or Los Angeles, that sigh of relief you offer to the gods probably came originally from air almost as bad. Many cities with populations above 500,000 have serious pollution problems. Consider the sulfur dioxide alone in city air. It causes nylon hosiery to disintegrate; it erodes marble and granite. The skin's systems can scarcely be treated more charitably. Along a waterfront or within short walking distance of a factory that uses chemicals (so many do), the harsh, toxic gases that get into the air make matters much worse.

City Skin appears to find a special target in women over forty, though it does not wholly spare men and women who are younger than that.

The condition shows up in a number of ways—redness, dryness, discoloration, and spots on the skin. The symptoms are deceptive, for they often resemble those of seborrhea, acne, psoriasis, or some elusive contact dermatitis—and maybe all of them.

In my consulting rooms it becomes difficult not to associate City Skin with the increasing number of patients who come in with pyogenic dermatoses (those with pus formations), seborrhea of the scalp (the excessive oiliness from which severe dandruff usually develops), and folliculitis (inflammation of the hair follicles).

But all these itemized melancholy consequences of city living relate mainly to pollutants that make a direct assault on the skin. The floating gases and aerial debris that sensitize the skin and bring about allergic reactions are even more numerous. The observant dermatologist must first discover whether there is a relationship to air pollution. If so, a protective, healing cream is prescribed and the patient is advised to avoid contaminated atmosphere. It should come as no surprise that the best way to avoid City Skin is to try to stay out of the city air when the smog is excessive. Absurdly obvious, of course, and impractical.

But there are a number of self-help measures that can be taken both to avoid and to heal City Skin. The dual goal is to protect the skin from the noxious air and to adopt measures that will maintain your gains once you've begun to shield your skin from the city atmosphere.

Since sunshine is a major part of the problem, begin by protecting a sun-sensitive skin with cosmetics containing sunshielding agents; some examples are Reflecta®, Sun Block®, Uval®, and Solebar®.

Wash regularly and often with a bar-type neutral or pure soap containing a recognized antiseptic for the skin. Recommended is a nonirritating soap. Before making up, women should use a moisturizing cream; it will leave a thin layer of emollient. After removing the makeup at night, give the face and adjoining exposed surfaces a quick treatment with a cleansing or detergent cream; it will remove the impacted soot and grime as well as soften the skin. Then apply an astringent and gently pat on moisturizing cream again. Men should wash thoroughly at night to rinse all traces of noxious elements, followed by the use of a healing or moisturizing cream.

Because of the drying effect of City Skin, lines tend to form on the skin areas exposed all day. The lines, which should be caught early, are best handled by a soft vegetable cream massaged on face, eyelids, forehead, and neck.

In private practice I have been treating City Skin as a single, unified complex of skin disorders brought on by a variety of assaults, rather than approaching one or two of its more prominent component disorders, I have therefore been obliged to seek a more direct treatment than a simple cosmetic can provide.

For that reason I have experimentally formulated a protective cream intended to work as both a preventive and a remedy for City Skin. Since it is still experimental and subject to a good deal of further study, it would serve no purpose to publish the formula, though I am gratified by its performance thus far. Its main components, however, are a moisturizer to avoid dryness and to lubricate the skin, a fluid silicone to act as a chemical barrier against the atmospheric vandals, a sunscreening agent, another ingredient (incidentally a relative of allantoin) that stimulates and heals, emulsifiers that have a softening effect, and Vitamins A and D.

The cream is cosmetically acceptable because it is immediately absorbed into the skin without staining garments or bed linen. Twenty-six patients who have complained of smarting, irritation, burning, and blotching—a combination of quite classical symptoms of City Skin—were given the cream for daily use and reported rapid healing as well as a high degree of prevention of further outbreaks.

13

Your Skin in Winter

If summer and its drying sun are rough on skin, winter is no bargain either. Indeed, it requires more elaborate skin care measures.

You've heard it often:

"Out where we live, the temperature in midwinter often goes to zero or lower—but the air is so dry you'd never know it."

That dryness might deceive the sensory nerves just below the outer epidermal skin layer that distinguish between warm and cool, but the top layer is meanwhile quietly losing the moisture which makes for supple skin.

For it is "moisture" that is the magic word underlying the maintenance of a trouble-free skin in winter.

In summer, it is true that the skin is afflicted by the hazard of sunburn and on the beach harassed by breezes that are sometimes parching. But the summer is marked in most parts of the country by high relative humidity too— the quality in the atmosphere that contributes so greatly to the season's discomfort.

So far as the skin is concerned, that high humidity is the summer's saving grace. It is the skin's major protector against the aridity of the sun.

Even in those parts of the country where the prevailing winter humidity is high enough to make the cold seem colder than the temperature suggests, it is still lower than the summer's humidity reading, and the winds are sharper and more drying than in summer.

The skin distress of winter is worsened, of course, by our superheated homes. It does not help much that we are turning increasingly to heating systems that are called "winter air conditioning"—which is a more sophisticated form of old-fashioned "hot-air heat"—and abandoning the old steam radiator that so often, in its kindly, wheezing way, leaked enough steam into the room to keep the humidity at an advantageous level.

Living, as most of us do, in zones with fast-changing weather conditions, you can't win 'em all, but your skin can at least break even if you will take the measures necessary every day to help it survive until spring. Otherwise, March 21 may find your outer surface in a condition that suggests the reason for the expression "alligator skin."

It is easier to understand what needs to be done if you realize that the skin's outermost layer should contain about 15 percent water, and when that percentage falls below 10 the skin becomes noticeably dry. The body's own defense against such dryness is the natural oil, sebum, that it constantly produces to keep the skin lubricated and soft. The sebum, of course, also gives some moisture back to the skin from which it came. Perspiration does it too, of course, but that is a scarce wintertime commodity except, fortunately, in those superheated living quarters.

To maintain an effective balance between the skin and the moisture level it requires, the relative humidity should not be over 60 percent; above that the excess moisture in the air will be absorbed by the skin. That is unlikely to be harmful to beauty; the usually attractive skin of British women is generally attributed to their country's moist climate.

In our highly heated homes, the humidity level is frequently no higher than 20 percent, often 15. At such low levels, the moisture in the skin's outer layer is transpired into the room's atmosphere faster than it is replaced. The act of simply moving about also contributes to evaporation. It also is evident that some skins tend to dry out more than others do; therefore, the owner of a customarily "dry" skin must take more stringent measures than usual.

First, consider exposure to the outdoors. Avoid all the assault by wind and cold that is possible by covering up to the eyes, and protect the face and hands. Before leaving home in markedly cold weather, rub an emollient cream into the skin areas that will be exposed—the nose, cheeks, and forehead, as well as the ears if they are going to be exposed. Makeup can be applied over the moisturizing cream.

A moisturizer usually consists of a cream or lotion emulsified in water or oil; it may also contain lanolin or cholesterol, vitamins, hormones, stearic acid, triethanolamine, and perfume. Penetrating agents, exotic fragrances and oils, a natural moisture fraction, and herbal extracts can also be added. Nothing put on a dry skin should contain alcohol, so read all labels carefully.

Inside the home, or even an office, ascertain whether there is some sort of humidification provided. There may not be much you can do about it in an office over which you have no control, except perhaps for placing a shallow vessel on or under a radiator and keeping some water in it.

Hot-air heating systems are, as noted, especially drying and should have a built-in evaporator that moisturizes the air as it comes up from the furnace. If yours doesn't have it, the cost of installing one would be warranted by health considerations, not only with respect to benefits to the skin but also for prevention of respiratory ailments.

Bathing takes a little extra care in cold weather because the warm water has several effects. It dissolves the protective oil film, permitting the skin's moisture to escape after the towel-drying. Also, the warm water and the normal rubbing of the bathing action remove with the grime just

enough of the top skin layer to expose a more porous surface. Thus, the bath should be converted from a drying
experience to a lubrication job. Bath oils can be added to
the water.

Bath oils contain mineral or vegetable oils such as
sesame, olive, or avocado; an emulsifier such as isopropyl
myristate, solubilized lanolin, or sterols, and perfume.
When one teaspoonful is placed in the bath water, the bath
fluid becomes milky and fragrant. Small microscopic oil
droplets and fragrance adhere to the skin and make the
bather feel like Cleopatra or Raquel Welch. A bath oil can
be helpful softening and perfuming the skin and leaving it
thinly oil-coated. Some bath oils have a dispersing action so
that they are not only a plus for the skin but also act as a
water softener. For those who prefer the shower there are
many oils available to spray on afterward.

The bath soap should not be highly alkaline because
that, too, removes the natural oil film and diminishes the
acid mantle that protects the skin.

Washing the skin gently—no sturdy rubbing is needed—
with a soft washcloth or a natural or synthetic sponge not
only cleanses but also offers a massage helpful to the
circulation. Towel-drying should be done gently.

After drying, massage the entire body with a good skin
lotion or emollient cream, giving special attention to such
problem areas as the heels, knees, hands, and elbows. Bath
or not, give yourself the same emollient treatment before
bed and upon arising daily. You may have special areas that
need emollient emphasis, such as the sides of the ankles,
heels, or soles.

Use a moisturizing cream at least once daily; if that is
all the time you can spare, make it in the morning and take
some special pains with the face and throat because of
their greater exposure to the elements outside. The skin is
hydrated by the moisturizer except for an invisible surface

film that retards evaporation of moisture from the skin and, incidentally, offers a good base for foundation makeup.

As I noted at the outset, the key word in maintaining good skin health through the winter is "moisture," and it is a quality that must be diligently protected from evaporation by the regular application of familiar types of oils and creams that keep it from literally blowing away in the wind.

For one who engages in winter outdoor sports the challenge to the skin is greatly multiplied. The protective measures noted above must be doubled, and protective lotions applied more frequently. In addition, of course, the lips must be protected with a special lipstick to prevent chapping and, most important, a summer-type suntan lotion or cream should be applied every few hours to thwart the special treachery of the sun in the wintertime.

14

Skin Hygiene for Travelers

The cosmetic routines you practice at home can easily be continued when you're off on vacation. The hygienic routines *must* be—only more so. As to both, you *can* take them with you.

On holidays abroad we submit the skin, the body, and the stamina to far more demands than usual even without considering the added strains of a strange physical environment, the time-change shock, and the sudden imposition of another culture's discipline (multiplied by the number of countries visited). We often encounter the frustrations of a language barrier and, almost always, unaccustomed diets.

Obviously, the traveler needs a good capacity for easy psychological and physical adjustments. If you can make them with the smooth shifting of an automatic transmission, travel is for you. If your body and spirit respond to such changes with the reluctance of a balky gear lever, you'll be happier spending those first two weeks of July at a picnic ground within easy walking distance.

Vacationing anywhere means that your skin will experience the effects of more walking, more sun exposure, more road dust or train soot, often more wind and, if you are camping, an abundance of less controllable hazards.

Traveling in Western Europe and America, you will

meet in most places few shortages of the facilities and products you want. But in isolated regions, and more surely outside the country, you will have more trouble finding such amenities as the kinds of bathing facilities, health products, and cosmetics to which you are accustomed.

Because foreign travel attracts more tourists every year, hotels abroad are coming to meet the demand for the kind of private bathing facilities we have at home. Take along these home-produced cosmetics you need or may want. In choosing them you will learn, perhaps to your surprise, how few are real necessities.

Except for liquids, put all your cosmetics in plastic, break-resistant containers, the kind drugstores use for pills. For free-flowing liquids, use soft plastic containers with screw caps sealed tightly with cellophane tape; in a plane your luggage goes into a nonpressurized baggage compartment where the lower atmospheric pressure causes liquids to leak. Even better than carrying cosmetics in plastic containers is to get them in stick form, and many of them are now made that way.

If a difference in soaps has ever caused you a problem at home, carry your own brand abroad with you. Should you have some special sensitivity about toilet tissue, take along a roll or two of your own.

Make a point of getting bath or shower facilities as you move about; if they are not as private as you'd like, take them anyway. Bathing is of special importance to your feet, which take most of the vacation's punishment, so soak them each night, dry carefully between the toes, push back the cuticles, and keep the toenails well trimmed. If calluses form on the feet, remove or reduce them with a pumice stone, working it gently and prudently to avoid causing more trouble than you prevent.

The most important solution for foot problems is a pair of suitable walking shoes (with changeovers); you may be losing some fashion value but you'll be gaining a happier vacation. Summer-type shoes—toeless or backless—could be a disaster. High heels are not only tiring but also tend to get wedged between cobblestones, which are still common abroad. Even on flat pavements they are unsuitable.

By all means, carry in your purse the suntan lotion that works best for you at home, and use it frequently. A disabling sunburn at home is a real nuisance; on vacation it could be tragic. (See Chapter 8, on sunburn and tanning.)

Also purse-toted at all times should be some packets of dry-wash, very handy when out-of-hotel cleansing is needed. With it might be carried a small quantity of witch hazel for a skin freshening wherever you may be; almost any foreign pharmacy will have it.

For the winter holiday on skis, which is becoming so popular, skin care is not only advisable but also urgent. Wind has a severe and painful chapping effect, and sunlight reflected from white snow poses the same sunburn hazard at below freezing as sunlight does on a beach in August. Thus, the skier should use a suntan lotion or cream; in addition, emollient creams are especially beneficial.

What to Take Along

In deciding on what to take along and what to buy while traveling, a matter of economics arises; availability, too. If the manufacturers also make their products in foreign plants, the quality is standard and price is likely to be low. If a product must be imported it will be quite costly—and scarce.

Below is a list of what else to take with you, in addition to the products mentioned above. The list at first glance might suggest a mini-drugstore, but they are all small items that will pack compactly. Assemble them well in advance rather than during pre-takeoff fever to avoid mid-trip panic as you begin to wonder whether you packed the cobra-venom antidote. Label everything legibly and explicitly. Now pop in:

Antimicrobial skin ointment (for minor cuts, burns, infections)

Calamine lotion (for sunburn, windburn, itch, dermatitis)

Antiseptic soap (for cleansing abraded skin)

Tweezers (for plucking splinters, etc.)

Antifungal skin ointment (especially for the tropics)

Zinc Undecylenate foot powder (for daily dusting to protect against fungi, other infections)

Band-Aids, three-inch elastic bandage, two-inch gauze bandages, four-by-four-inch gauze pads

Adhesive tape, Scotch tape

Insect repellent (imperative in the tropics)

A few further travel hints are vital though not skin-related:

• Diarrhea, or dysentery, often strikes tourists abroad (where it is known generically as *la turista*). Carry Kaopectate, Donnagel, or paregoric, though nearly all foreign countries have devised quite effective remedies out of bitter experience.

• For drugs you must take regularly, as prescribed by your doctor, carry a few extra prescriptions rather than just one if you will be moving around.

• If you use drugs abroad that your doctor has not prescribed, bring back the labels so that he will know what you've been taking.

• Carry an extra pair of your prescription glasses. And, just in case, an extra prescription for them.

• Purchase directory with names of doctors who speak English.

Remedies on the Run

There are other possible afflictions that go with travel, but coping with them all by medically accepted techniques would require that you take along a small hospital dispensary and some operating-room equipment. Lacking them, the vacationer might do worse than heed the counsel of Dr. Peter Horvath, clinical professor of medicine and chief of dermatology at Georgetown University Medical Center, Washington, D.C. For the traveler-in-motion he suggests these practical, *al fresco* remedies:

Sunburn. Apply sour cream or yogurt. They cool the burn and relieve the smarting. Lukewarm baths with non-perfumed bath oil will also help.

Jellyfish stings. If applied within ten to fifteen minutes, a paste of meat tenderizer works fine. It neutralizes the poison. Good also for Portuguese man-of-war stings.

Insect bite (ordinary). Drugstore nonprescription anesthetic cream products suppress the itching. A hot compress is also helpful.

Bee, hornet, and similar stings. Ice is safest. If sting is severe, or lingers beyond twelve hours, see a doctor. Don't try to remove an imbedded stinger lest serious infection result. It will disintegrate in time.

Ticks. Try to coax the tick to withdraw by touching it with a lighted match or cigarette. Breaking off its head will invite infection.

15

The Pill Can Affect
Your Skin–and Hair

We are now well into the second decade since the Pill made its dramatic debut as the most novel and effective means of contraception ever devised. Its effects, as well as the implications for the future control of a dangerously expanding population, are sweeping.

The Pill's effectiveness and its availability have combined to force a secondary result long overdue—the abandonment by states, nations, and religious sects of their age-old bans against contraception as a matter of personal choice. Not all these forces have yet relented, but the pressures will in time prove irresistible.

As of now, probably more than nine million American women use the Pill regularly and when some outstanding doubts about its total safety have been removed, as they will be, the number will continue to grow. When it was first introduced on a broad scale, it was known that the long-range effects were not entirely predictable and that it would take perhaps twenty years to be sure. We are now well past the midway mark for that period and, while some problems have indeed arisen, their frequency leaves the early confidence in the Pill largely intact.

Basically, what makes the Pill work is that it causes the female reproductive system to imitate pregnancy. In true pregnancy, the process of ovulation ceases—that is, there is no monthly release from the ovary of an egg (ovum), which exposes it to fertilization; otherwise, a woman three months pregnant could conceive again and begin to develop a second embryo, thereby delivering two babies three months apart. Nature logically ensures against that.

The Pill contains, essentially, a combination of synthetic female hormones, estrogen and progesterone, which are taken separately or together. The estrogens are the hormones that truly separate the girls from the boys, for it is these that impart such distinctively female characteristics as the breasts, the unique female figure, and the usually higher voice. Progesterone regulates the menstrual cycle and sees to the nourishment of the fertilized egg in the early phase of pregnancy.

Side effects from the use of the Pill were recognized immediately upon its introduction. In some cases there was nausea or vomiting—which is expected as a usual accompaniment of an early pregnancy—but the most frequent was water retention, which caused an increase in weight and an uncomfortable sense of heaviness of the breasts. These symptoms usually vanish after a few months of use.

However, the most disturbing development was the occurrence of cases of thrombophlebitis associated with using the Pill. This clotting within the blood vessels, usually in the legs or feet, can have grave implications, but the occurrence was not frequent enough statistically to be confirmed as a widespread threat.

Some of these consequences were diminished with the development of a "sequential" pill, in which the order of the use of the hormones has been rearranged. The first fifteen tablets, one taken each day beginning six days after menstruation ceases, contain only estrogen. The last five tablets taken in the cycle contain both estrogen and progesterone. Different manufacturers vary their formulas somewhat for the purpose of avoiding side effects, but basically their products rely upon the two types of hormones.

It should be noted in fairness that some suspicions have been raised about a possibly higher frequency of uterine cancer among Pill users, but the statistical evidence on that score is incomplete. At the time of this writing, one scientific investigator has reported experimental success in reducing that hazard with a Pill into which a new hormone element has been introduced.

Not all of the Pill's reported side effects have been unhappy ones. Some previously infertile women who had used the Pill for a time reported that they had become joyfully pregnant after stopping its use. Also, physicians have found that in many instances the Pill was directly helpful in correcting menstrual irregularity (amenorrhea), excessive flow (menorrhagia), or excessive pain (dysmenorrhea). It was having a widespread psychological benefit too by improving gratification in the sex act for many couples for whom gratification had previously been limited because of tension due to the fear of pregnancy.

Striking benefits, moreover, are achieved by older women, those who have entered menopause and do not need the Pill for contraceptive purposes; for them, the Pill's estrogen compensates for the waning of its natural production, helps to relieve distressing menopausal symptoms, and bridges gracefully the abrupt gap between middle age and old age. In this case, however, a special formulation of the Pill is required and it must be prescribed and supervised by an expert gynecologist. The subject is discussed in greater detail in Chapter 16, under the broader topic of hormone use.

The Pill's effect on the skin, however, has varied from favorable to unfavorable, although the favorable consequences are more common, due to the basic fact that a woman's production of estrogen, as a natural process of being feminine, is what gives her a fairer skin than the male's.

There is also a central contradiction in the relationship

of the Pill and the skin. Dr. John Strauss of Boston has observed that estrogen has the effect of reducing the flow of sebum, the body's natural oil. As we have seen, it is the excessive flow of sebum, which comes up through the sebaceous ducts in the skin, that encourages the familiar infections that first take the form of whiteheads, which soon turn into blackheads, pustules, and even cysts. When such an outbreak gets out of control, the condition is acne, the most common of skin disorders.

Since the most helpful thing that can happen in most cases of acne is a reduction in the flow of sebum, the Pill and its estrogen content promise—on the basis of results already noted by Dr. Strauss—to become an important part of the overall therapy for acne. It seems especially effective in treating acne among older-age groups although—and here is the contradiction—their natural production of sebum is already diminishing.

Of the side effects attending the normal use of the Pill that have come to my notice in dermatological practice, the case I recall best involved a young woman of twenty-six who had come to me with a severe case of papular cystic acne. She had acne even before she began to use the Pill sixteen months earlier. The Pill had done her facial condition no good; in addition, four months before her visit to my office she had developed deep, irregular, brownish pigment patches on her cheeks and forehead.

As mentioned earlier, this unsightly pigmentation, a well-known side effect of the Pill, is called chloasma. It is popularly known less precisely as the "mask of pregnancy" and as "liver spots," although the liver has nothing to do with it. The condition appears most commonly on the cheeks and forehead. In the case of this patient, an alternate contraceptive method was recommended and a pigment-reducing cream took care of the pigment patches. Healing the acne took a bit longer, but it was eventually cleared up by the available treatments.

There is also believed to be a relationship between use of the Pill and the growth of hair. In looking at that situation it is necessary to take into account not only the female hormones but also the basic male hormone, testosterone. Just as normal women secrete a small quantity of testosterone, normal men also produce minor quantities of the female hormone.

A fundamental point to remember is that, just as the female hormones seem quite clearly to be responsible for the woman's smooth, soft, and abundant hair, it has been quite clearly demonstrated that excessive testosterone secretion can be the cause of baldness. Surely, we are confronted by the superficial consideration that far more men than women go bald, although there are other evidences that support a cause-and-effect relationship between testosterone and thinning hair.

One of them is the conspicuous fact that women who show excessive hair loss may also show masculine characteristics, indicating excessive production of testosterone. These are frequently women who, like balding men, may show excessive hair growth on other parts of the body, which is an unfortunate paradox.

Since the Pill's introduction, dermatologists have been noting a growing rate of hair loss by women, but that is more or less a general observation in which the Pill has not been specifically pinpointed as the cause. It is my own suspicion that in the period since the Pill's introduction there have been a number of coinciding medical and cosmetic developments that might as easily be blamed for the hair loss.

Further study of a Pill-baldness relationship, if any, seems to be warranted by a set of observations advanced by Dr. Frank Cormia of the Cornell University Medical College in New York.

He observed that some women who have been on the Pill for an extended period of time do indeed show hair thinning—but it begins, as a rule, *a month or so after they have stopped taking the Pill.* The same thing happens to women *after* they have delivered a baby.

Dr. Cormia reasoned that since pregnancy increases production of the female hormones, which appear to prevent baldness in women, the Pill must also have the same effect because it keeps the hormone level high. Therefore, when she abandons use of the Pill, a woman is likely to have similar post-pregnancy symptoms, and it happens in this way:

There is always a regular process of normal hair loss—actually a cycle of growth, loss, and regrowth. But during pregnancy (or use of the Pill) it seems to be the "loss" phase that is largely suspended. When the pregnancy ends (or use of the Pill is interrupted) the cycle goes back to normal, but it starts with the "loss" phase that has been missed. It takes time to catch up with the others.

Dr. Cormia offered the comforting assurance that the condition is only temporary, and while going off the Pill might cause some initial hair thinning, the growth cycle will be normal again in six months or so, and certainly in less than a year if the process of hormone production is normal.

As I have noted, there are other possible causes of rising hair loss among women that have appeared in the past decade or so, coinciding with the Pill's advent. A physician consulted by a woman with thinning hair must learn from her how long she has been taking the Pill, whether she has abandoned it, how many children she has had, and when the last was born. Has she had menstrual irregularity (a possible clue to a glandular disorder, which might also cause hair loss)? Is there an iron deficiency? Has she been taking pills or other medication known possibly to cause hair thinning, such as amphetamine pills, perhaps amphetamine or Dexedrine for "reducing," or tranquilizers or other sedatives?

Does she use hair straightener or "tease" her hair? Or a too-stiff bristle hairbrush, a nylon hairbrush, or brush rollers? They can all encourage loss of hair. So, too, can heparin, an anticoagulant used by heart patients, or some of the anticholesterol drugs. Discontinuing all of these will soon show results.

Obviously, the doctor must look for evidence of scalp disease. Or the self-imposed, irresistible traction of the ponytail or other tight hairdo.

Any of these factors might exist concurrently with the use of the Pill and might be the true cause of the hair problem.

The introduction of the Pill has brought blessings to millions of women. Besides its value as a superior, more dependable contraceptive method, the Pill helps to regulate irregular periods and improves the smoothness of the skin. Together with these signal benefits, however, have come certain attendant disadvantages for perhaps 20 percent of women who use the Pill, including blood clots, dizziness, nausea, and increased, sometimes blotchy skin pigmentation. A woman should be alert to any such physical change while she is using the Pill and report it promptly to her doctor. So far medical science has not discovered any method whereby the doctor can determine in advance whether a woman is one of the happy 80 percent or the less fortunate 20 percent. Perhaps in time we shall learn how to distinguish. Meanwhile, the most important fact is in most cases the advantages of this great modern discovery far outweigh the disadvantages.

16

Hormones, Hair, and Easing the Change of Life

Like all apocryphal stories that are durable, the reputed episode in the French Chamber of Deputies (or was it the Senate?) has varied in details as it has passed from generation to generation. The Deputy (or Senator) had the floor and was pleading eloquently for (or against) a proposed measure that may (or may not) have been concerned with fixing maximum working hours for women. At one point he felt obliged to emphasize a distinction that had probably not escaped his colleagues' notice.

". . . for, as between men and women," he observed, "there is a difference."

The Chamber came to its feet and, as one man, shouted with fervor:

"Vive la différence!"

That response denoted grateful recognition of a fact, but not an understanding of why it was so.

It is the sex hormones that make *la différence:* the female hormones, estrogen and progesterone, and the male hormone, testosterone.

And whether you are of one sex or the other—or even undecided—these glands and hormones can make or break your skin, and your hair too. That holds for both men and women, although the influence may be somewhat more decisive for women because they have the capacity for bear-

178

ing children; the female glandular system is therefore more complex and, it follows, more subject to imbalance.

A baby girl, diapered, can seldom be distinguished from a baby boy. Although their primary sex organs differ, if their mothers do not give them distinctive dress and hair styles they would perhaps have to be four or five years old before they could be identified by sex. By that time they are taking separate paths toward manhood and woman-hood, but not until their early teens do they become full members of their sexes. The sex glands then become operative, but being new at the job, they often overdo it. By an intricate process, they stimulate the glands that produce sebum. The oil ducts become plugged, resulting in the formation of pimples, pustules, abscesses, and cysts. If the condition gets out of control, as it often does, we have another adolescent with acne, a condition discussed in detail in Chapter 3.

The sex hormones, as soon as they are activated, present problems that have nothing to do with their intended func-tion of reproduction. Fortunately, as a rule, they soon settle down to that primary purpose. Normally, they pose no further difficulties until about one's fortieth birthday or later. At that age a man—with a rather simple sexual design and outlook—still has a decade or two of reproductive ca-pacity remaining, though his interest in the subject is not what it was fifteen or twenty years earlier. It's just that his sex mechanism is getting a bit tired, though he may not believe it.

For a woman at that age, *la différence* is showing again, and unhappily so. Nature has ordained that her reproduc-tive years are over and it begins to neglect her. As she enters menopause, she is relieved of the basic mission of reproduc-tion. Menstruation ceases, for which she is probably grate-ful. No longer a child bearer, she has far less need for those marvelous estrogen and progesterone hormones, so their production begins to dwindle.

The tiny oil glands under the skin now supply sebum more sparingly and even the perspiration glands become less active as production is reduced. The oil and perspiration, until now, have blended on the skin, lubricating it, keeping it soft and attractive. With those lubricants now less abundant, the skin is drier and in warm weather may become hot and flushed. Tiny lines form on the forehead and at the corners of the eyes, a portent of the wrinkles to come later.

Now, on the upper lip and elsewhere on the face, a fuzz of colorless lanugo hairs appears; not only have the shrinkage of the skin and its increasing thinness made the hairs more evident than they had been before, but also the reduction in the flow of the female hormones, which tend to keep the woman's face free of hair, has been aggravated by the greater relative dominance of the male hormones that all women produce to a minor extent. It is the male hormones that grow facial hair; at least that is the dominant belief. Probably for this same reason the scalp hair, after menopause begins, becomes thinner, sparser, drier, and rather lifeless.

The matter of excessive hair where it is not wanted—and a deficit where it ought to be—is given a more troublesome dimension if the adrenal gland, situated just above the kidney, becomes overactive and causes the secretion of too much of what is not needed—the male-related hormone androgen.

Serious and knowledgeable dermatologists have come up with a score of reasons to explain the common pattern type of baldness, and while none of them has been persuasive enough to exclude all the other possibilities, all seem logical enough to warrant consideration. But perhaps the most impressive results have come from an experiment directed by Dr. J. B. Hamilton, an imaginative hair researcher at the University of the State of New York Downtown Medical Center in Brooklyn. Although the experiment was conducted about two decades ago, no one has since challenged its findings convincingly.

Dr. Hamilton fortunately had access to more than one hundred eunuchoids, males who had been castrated for medical reasons at various ages (it makes a difference at what stage of sexual development a male ceases to produce the androgens). Hair growth ranged from very thin to at least good; none was balding. For a random group, sharing only the single characteristics of sex impairment, the fact that none showed signs of advanced hair thinning was in itself remarkable.

Each of the castrates was regularly given doses of testosterone, which is probably the most potent of the male hormones. In a relatively short time, most of them began to show receding hairlines or other scalp hair loss. When the testosterone was withdrawn, all of them had regrowth back to normal.

Banishing Unwanted Hair

Superfluous hair can, of course, be handled routinely, but the procedure becomes endless. There are chemical depilatories sold over drugstore counters, but they can be pretty harsh on some skins and, anyway, the hair growth returns in a week or two. The rip-it-off approach entails spreading warm wax over the hair and, when it cools and hardens, stripping the wax off in a single, quick swipe with the hope that the hairs have become imbedded in the hardened wax, which should take them along. The simplest method, of course, is using a safety razor—fast and safe but least enduring. (It is not true that shaving speeds hair regrowth.) At least, the razor is less painful than the wax stripping.

The most effective method of depilation is electrolysis, in which an electric needle is inserted into the hair follicle, coagulates the hair bulb, and scars the papilla so that the follicle will not again produce hair. The operation requires great skill and an extremely sensitive touch, and must be performed by an electrologist of known competence to avoid some possible hazards. It requires much more patience and more money than the other methods do, but a skilled operator can remove hair permanently, even if some stubborn hairs need two or three assaults. Over the long run, electrolysis might even prove to be less costly than repeated home treatments with other methods.

The only thing a dermatologist can do directly with regard to hirsutism, which is excessive and undesirable hair growth, is to prescribe hormones and steroids, taken by mouth, that will depress the activity of the adrenal secretions and therefore the androgen production. A dermatologist who rejects that approach should not be pressed; he is likely to have good reason for it. The results are commonly poor.

Hormone Creams

I remain open-minded about the hormonal and steroid creams for which, when used by hormone-deficient women whose skin is beginning to show it, restorative powers are claimed. The superficial amount of estrogen and progesterone in cosmetic hormone creams, when used for long periods of time, may have a slight favorable effect. When used externally in therapeutic doses, the hormone creams may soften the lines but not remove the wrinkles completely, because of the pathology under the deep tissues of the skin.

At a meeting of the Cosmetic Chemists some years ago, Dr. E. Silson reported favorable effects on the skin of a cream containing the steroid pregnenolone. Half of the face was used as a control. No side effects were noted. An article in the *Journal of the American Medical Association*, however, cites a case of unusual menstrual bleeding after excessive use of hormone cream. In this case, the patient used large doses of a cream containing estrogen too frequently, without medical supervision.

Recently, a foreign cosmetic company placed on the market a substitute for collagen, the tissue under the skin that gives it firmness. They claim this will smooth out lined skin. Only time will tell. Some years ago in Germany, a cosmetic cream containing large doses of placental extract was marketed with the enthusiastic claims that it made the skin look youthful. In the United States the Food and Drug Administration ordered this product removed from the American cosmetic market for lack of any substantial proof of the accuracy of its manufacturers' claims.

Is there any dependable method for slowing almost completely the aging process in the skin? Dr. Robert Wilson is convinced that there is. Dr. Wilson is a respected gynecologist who also practices endocrinology, the branch of medicine that relates to the more common glands. He is the founder of the Wilson Research Foundation, which is deeply concerned with means of arresting the painful symptoms of the aging process in women, and is respected by the medical profession.

A few years ago Dr. Wilson published *Feminine Forever!*, a definitive book about his theories and his results in applying them. Essentially, the volume documents his unshakable belief that menopause is entirely unnecessary. It can be avoided, he maintains, if a woman—preferably when about to enter menopause—begins a regimen that centers on taking estrogen cyclically. Specifically, it would be taken daily for twenty-one days, followed by seven days when it is not taken. The total of twenty-eight days, it will be noted, corresponds to the menstrual cycle, and Dr. Wilson believes that menstruation will then continue unabated for virtually the rest of the woman's life! (She will, however, become infertile at about the usual age.)

The Wilson doctrine has a simple central theme: if the

artificial estrogen takes up the slack caused by the dwindling of the natural estrogen supply, the menopause simply never happens and life goes on pretty much as before. The hormone routine, this theory maintains, should be continued even into the nineties!

Among the many hundreds of patients whose estrogen cycle he has prescribed and supervised, Dr. Wilson reports the following observations:

Menstrual periods may continue normally. The sudden hot flashes and the nervous spells of menopause vanish. The skin feels and looks more plump and elastic instead of hollowing and sagging. The patient is cheerful and easy to live with, rather than a neurotic bundle of woe to husband and family. The sex urge remains at a high level. Periods of depression are reduced markedly, and perhaps as important as any other benefit, the woman retains and continues to pursue the same values, goals, and activities that always were for her the essence of living.

It cannot be too strongly stressed that this regimen must be prescribed and closely supervised by a gynecologist or a family doctor who is familiar with the procedure, just as the regular use of the contraceptive Pill—which the cyclical estrogen closely resembles—must be. There are still some outstanding suspicions about a possible relationship between the regular use of sex hormones and uterine cancer. Surely, no doctor would permit either of these routines for a woman who, for example, had previously had uterine cancer or had a family history of it.

It also is necessary to determine, first, whether a woman requires estrogen therapy at all and, if so, whether the hormone should be taken by mouth or by injection. A good deal depends on the level of maturity of the natural estrogen in the blood serum. A number of tests have been devised to make this determination. For a long time the one used was known as the "17-ketosteroids" test. The test also exposed the presence of ovarian and adrenal tumors.

More sophisticated tests for blood-serum estrogen followed, and quite recently a much improved and very simple test has been devised.

An applicator swabs the vaginal wall and brings out a smear that is viewed by microscope, revealing what is called the estrogen maturation factor. It also permits a forecast of future estrogen activity. What is desirable is a high level of maturity and, if the need is indicated, estrogen therapy encourages this.

This test is helpful, to cite one example, in revealing whether the onset of wrinkling of the patient's face is due to an estrogenic deficiency or to some external cause, such as a compulsive habit of frowning, squinting, pouting, weeping—even smiling. Also, as described recently in *Annals of Internal Medicine*, wrinkles may be aggravated by smoking.

The new test is especially advantageous because the modern doctor uses the same sample for a Pap Test for possible uterine cancer, thus eliminating one troublesome trip to his surgery. In this test a cervical smear is taken and examined to determine the presence or absence of cancer cells. Should any be detected treatment can then be started without delay.

Not only women are concerned with the menopause and its consequences to skin, hair, nerves, spirit, and general sense of well-being. Many urologists and endocrinologists now believe that the male undergoes an equivalent period, though it may occur a few years later in life than for most women. The man, it is reported, shows anxiety, a depression neurosis, and a loss of personal drive that may even leave him reluctant to go to work every day. We have all probably noticed that men we know quite suddenly—although not always at the same ages—seem to age in facial appearance, weight, and general demeanor.

The cause of all this is the "change of life" syndrome, and it is probably brought on in men as it is in a woman by sudden waning of sex gland function. The condition is quite certain to be helped by injections of androgen, and more specifically, testosterone. The patient thereby risks a further advance of baldness, which must surely be already present to some degree, but by that time a bit of hair more or less may not matter much.

17

Dandruff–and How
to Abolish It

Dandruff is the product of excessive flow of scalp oil and is known clinically as *seborrhea capitis*. It has shown increasing incidence and severity in the past decade or so. As a medical problem it is rather more serious than most people realize; as a social problem it is rather less serious than we are being urged to believe.

Most people think of dandruff as being a hair problem. But dandruff originates on the scalp—which is part of the skin—and therefore cannot be separated from any consideration of skin problems.

Everyone has dandruff to some extent, and in moderate degree it is entirely normal. A certain quantity of scalp skin must constantly be flaking off in the process that is the skin's regular life cycle. Where the condition remains within normal bounds, the morning brushing or combing will handle the day's modest fallout quite adequately and it will probably not be noticed even by the scalp's owner.

When the condition becomes more than just a little snowy, "benign neglect" is probably not a benign solution. To clear this stubborn condition, a visit to your doctor or to a dermatologist could be time and money well spent.

The difficulty in treating this disorder is not that known causes are lacking but that they are too abundant. Also, two opposite skin conditions are related to dandruff: one is dry, the other greasy.

What is somewhat puzzling about dandruff is also the common age of occurrence. The body malfunctions related to it are so similar to those relating to acne, it would seem that they would occur simultaneously. While youngsters sometimes do have them together, it isn't often. Dandruff usually begins to show at about twenty, when acne has become a fading memory, and is not seen much after forty. (But if you get it after that it is not necessarily evidence of prolonged youth.) Within that age range about 80 percent of the population has it to a visible degree.

While the basic causes of seborrheic dandruff are not yet wholly clear, the behavioral and bacterial conditions that *stimulate* it are evident enough to make it generally possible to control it. The identified stimuli are internal and external. Prime attention must therefore be given to proper diet, essential hygiene, the correction of contributing constitutional problems, and effective external approaches.

The internal difficulties include an imbalance of hormones, poor general health or nutrition, dietary excesses with regard to fats, sugar, starch, and acid, and especially nervous tension. External triggers include chemical changes of the scalp's surface, increased volume and activity of the bacteria and fungi normally residing on the human scalp, an injury to the scalp, and inflammations that are reactions to the unwise use of cosmetics or topical medications.

The type of dandruff associated with a dry scalp is almost surely not the result of a bacterial infection but is more probably due to an abnormal and exaggerated bodily process known as too active keratinization.

One persuasive clue to the cause of dandruff has come from bacteriological studies that have consistently shown this: the scalp that is producing abundant dandruff is also the one giving shelter to an increased number of two bacterial and yeast organisms—*staphylococcus* and *pityrosporum ovale*. Clearing them reduces dandruff.

What we do know about dandruff is traceable to the fact that it is the most common of the scalp disorders, which has provided plenty of opportunity for observation and experiment.

It should be clear by now that dandruff itself is not a disease but only a symptom of one that is less visible and may be far more serious in terms of hair loss and possible baldness.

What Dandruff Is—and Does

The white, powdery patina observed on the shoulders of a dark suit or dress is not the only warning signal of dandruff. The scalp scales, and there is itching. In a man it may be accompanied by a progressive loss of hair, which can be observed on the comb, the hairbrush, and the bathroom sink. When the dandruff problem is at last overcome, the hair loss may stop; the lost hair may even be regrown. Then again, it may not.

The skin of the face may turn red and dry; the pores become enlarged and are covered with greasy scales. The big danger is that the relentless itching of the scalp will lead the distraught victim to dig the fingernails into it and scratch, either to relieve the itching or to remove the unsightly scales. The frequent result is a bacterial infection, which only multiplies the problem.

The discovery of dandruff flakes on parts of the body below the head does not necessarily mean they have dropped down from the hair. Seborrhea, and therefore dandruff, also afflict the eyebrows, chest, and outer surfaces of the ears, and they must be treated directly.

The seborrhea that goes with dandruff is substantially the same seborrhea that goes with acne; in both cases, the source is abnormal activity of the sebaceous glands that manufacture sebum. It seems beyond question that the leading cause of this dysfunction of the glands—though it is *not* the *only* cause—is the consumption of too much fat, especially animal. Fat taken into the body is normally used to build healthy tissue. But the body can use only so much fat; the excess goes often into unneeded weight, but there are limits even to that kind of use. The superexcess must be gotten rid of, so it is routed to the sebaceous glands as raw material for sebum.

The sebaceous glands secrete oil onto the skin as fast as it can be manufactured, and so it is the skin, scalp included, that is now stuck with the excess oil. Unless *washed away* about as fast as it collects, the oil continues to form a greasy scalp. The sebum and accumulated dust produce seborrhea. Resident bacteria flourish and may encourage further infection.

As if that weren't bad enough, another problem is added. It concerns the skin's protective acid mantle. In a healthy skin, the acid-alkali balance is tilted in favor of the acid side. Where dandruff is present, the acid mantle has been temporarily changed because the balance has shifted toward the alkali side. Therefore, a doctor treating a worse-than-usual case of dandruff is likely to prescribe acid-buffered cortisone liquid and shampoo for external application; they ease the itching, reduce flaking, and if other proper measures are taken, will help eradicate the dandruff.

People who are tense and show dandruff are especially difficult to treat. Not having the restraint that the scalp's itching and related discomforts demand, they will dig their fingernails into the scalp with special force, scoring it badly, drawing blood, and starting infections that often lead to folliculitis (inflammation of the hair follicles).

Blepharitis

It should be noted that the seborrhea that brings on dandruff has also been linked with a seriously inflamed condition of the eyelids known as *blepharitis.* Dr. C. Hickey has reported seborrhea present in a significant number of a group of two hundred blepharitis cases he has treated. Getting rid of the seborrhea, he has found, hastens the cure of the blepharitis. He cautioned that where both conditions exist together, special care must be taken when shampooing or showering to ensure that the infected debris from scalp and hair do not wash down onto the eyelids (to which I would add that the entire face should be similarly protected because it, too, is vulnerable). It can be done with a skin-tight waterproof shield that starts at the hairline. If the shower does not involve a shampoo, use of a tight shower cap will do.

Treating Dandruff

Effective treatment of dandruff-breeding scalp seborrhea includes mainly:

1. Shampooing regularly and, if the oily type, more frequently.
2. Application of antiseborrheic preparations, described below.
3. Scalp stimulation with ultraviolet or cold quartz rays.
4. Use of scalp lotions containing one or more of these ingredients: resorcinol, salicylic acid, quaternary amine, chloral hydrate, sulfur, or a mixture of these in a blend of water, alcohol, and glycerin.
5. Regular application of cortisone liquid preparations.

The *shampooing,* a form of scalp hygiene practiced regularly, will help greatly to control or even eradicate seborrheic dandruff that is not too far advanced. If the condition is moderate, over-the-counter remedies should also be tried

The regular shampoo is the most important remedy. If the scalp is not too oily, once a week may do; if oiliness is visible, shampooing twice a week, or more often, will be necessary. In general, keep the frequency just below the point where shampooing will bring on excessive dryness.

There are four general types of shampoos that are helpful; the choice may be dictated by trial and error because scalps react differently to each. They are:

Tincture of green soap is cleansing but contains a high proportion of alcohol that can dry hair and scalp with prolonged use. But dryness can be avoided by massaging a half-ounce of warm olive oil gently into the scalp right after shampooing.

Tar concentrate shampoo has a mild odor, is scale removing and cleansing, but continued use can cause contact dermatitis, a skin eruption, so watch it carefully.

Castile-and-olive-oil shampoo is the most popular of the four. Neutral, and probably safest of all because of its mildness, it contains coconut oil solution, dissolved flakes of Castile soap, and a little olive oil to prevent the dryness that the soap's high alkali content could cause. Because "Castile" is a term used loosely, purchase a well-known brand of good reputation.

There are also the *soapless detergent shampoos,* best used in cases of excessive oiliness. They do a fine cleansing job on the scalp, bringing out the hair's gloss and highlights. They, too, have a drying effect, the reason oily scalps like it. But if the shampoo dries too much, it should be followed directly by an olive oil massage of the scalp (not of the hair). If the drying effect is mild, the oil can be mixed with the shampoo as another ingredient. Use of an after-shampoo rinse containing quatenary amine is also helpful in neutralizing the soap and removing scales.

I might add parenthetically that I recently made a clinical evaluation of a shampoo containing biphenamine hydrochloride, Alvinine, and two containing zinc pyrithione, Zincon and Head and Shoulders, and found them effective against dandruff.

Your Pharmacist Can Help

If a popular brand of any of the above shampoos does not help—and switching types also does no good—your pharmacist should be able to formulate a good one. It can be supplemented for added effect by TBS or a similar antiseptic that is antibacterial and a deodorizer. For cosmetic value, the formula might also contain a soluble lanolin product such as isopropyl lanolin, which acts as an emollient and gives the hair a soft, glossy, healthy glow. Hair conditioners containing balsam and hydrolized protein build up the hair. If you've done your patient experimenting with all these formulas without a truly substantial effect on the dandruff, then seek out professional help. You need something with more muscle than shampooing alone. The choice and use of an antiseborrheic remedy requires the judgment and experience of a doctor.

Medication by Prescription

The most accepted antiseborrheic ointments contain sulfur, salicylic acid, resorcinol, and externally-used antiseptics. Your doctor will decide, but only after a proper diagnosis; then he must supervise your treatment.

The ointment or lotion is rubbed into the scalp nightly with the hair parted repeatedly to expose the scalp to the application—scalp, not hair.

Your doctor might suggest one of the newer dandruff formulas, some of which show much promise (and some are prescription-only products). These therapeutic medicated shampoos contain such ingredients as selenium sulfide, cadmium sulfide, zinc pyrithione, or captan, polythionates, bithionol, or allantoin complexes. All have been found very effective.

The medication is best kept on the scalp around the clock. For daytime use, a scalp-stimulating antiseptic hair lotion containing cortesone liquid and propylene glycol, such as Synalar®, Ficoid-5®, or Betnovate, will probably be most practical.

I have also been experimenting with a new product which seems effective in dandruff and hair fall. Evaluation tests are still continuing.

The Attack on All Fronts

Where dandruff is stubborn the resistance must be relentless. With proper shampooing and medication available, emphasis should turn to diet, a prime factor in seborrheic dandruff. The best kind of table manners will mean avoiding the seborrhea-inducing foods. As diets go, luckily, the one pertaining to seborrhea and dandruff does not demand maximum discipline. Following it will also be helpful to anyone suffering from other skin disorders, excess weight, or high blood pressure, although the diet in each case must be approached on its own special merits.

It was long believed by many physicians that diet was not a significant factor in cases of seborrhea. Independent support for my observations pointing to its importance came in 1971 from Dr. Wolfgang Caspar of St. Vincent's Medical Center in New York City, when he reported new findings regarding seborrhea of the skin and scalp at the International Conference of Dermatology in Venice in 1972. Dr. Caspar reported not only that improper diet leads to seborrhea, but also that seborrheic patients suffer from an easily disturbed carbohydrate metabolism with malabsorption or malutilization of Vitamin B_{12}. In cases of seborrhea it is advisable, therefore, to supplement the diet by taking Vitamin B_{12} orally or consulting a doctor, who may inject this vitamin. Local ultraviolet is also helpful.

The following is the diet I suggest for my seborrheic patients, whether the scalp or the face is involved:

SEBORRHEIC DIET

Avoid:

Excessive amounts of chocolate, iodized salt, shellfish, butter, spices, nuts, gooey desserts, and very hot coffee and tea. (Hot beverages dilate the capillaries of the nasal and cheek areas of the face.)

Use in Moderation:

Bacon, pork, ham, spicy cheese, fried and greasy foods, oils, ketchup, and pepper.

Eat Abundantly:

Lean meats, poultry, fish, low-fat milk, fruits, vegetables, salads, bread, sugar and salt substitutes, natural herbs, moderate amounts of salt.

18

Recognizing Common Skin Disorders

As the preceding chapters have shown, there is a great deal one can do to protect the health of his or her skin and to enhance its youthful and attractive appearance. Considering the complexity of its structure and functions, the skin is an organ that gives relatively little serious trouble for the greater part of our lives. There are times, however, when illness strikes the skin just as may happen to any other vital organ. When this occurs, the sooner the disquieting symptoms are checked by a doctor well versed in dermatology, and treatment is started, the better. Some skin diseases, such as herpes zoster, or shingles, can often be nipped in the bud by early treatment, but if neglected in the hope that they will "clear up by themselves" can quickly spread and become aggravated with painful and sometimes serious results.

It is important, therefore, to be familiar with the common skin disorders and their symptoms. Some of them, such as allergies and acne, have been discussed in other parts of this book. In this chapter, just to be forewarned and forearmed, let's look at some other skin ailments that can occur and that require the attention of your doctor. We shall briefly run through the more common ones and discuss their symptoms and treatment.

Psoriasis is a chronic skin disorder that usually affects the scalp, elbows, knees, chest, back, extremities, and nails. It is identified by the appearance of thick, whitish, adherent scales on a background of reddish patches. The patches may itch severely. On the nails, deep pits appear. In some cases only the nails are involved.

Treatment for psoriasis consists of the application of oils, creams, or ointments, which remove the scales. The most effective treatment known until recently was with preparations containing salicylic acid, tar, athralin, and allantoin. Today, however, dermatologists often treat psoriasis with salves containing derivatives of cortisone. Methotrexate, taken internally, is often prescribed for serious cases. Since methotrexate is a dangerous drug that has serious side effects, it must be used with caution and can only be obtained on the prescription of a doctor.

Impetigo is a pustular inflammation of the skin, which usually involves the cheeks. It is characterized by the appearance of yellow crusts and sores. The disease is highly contagious and may spread from one child to another in nurseries and schools. Treatment consists of washing away the scales with antiseptic soap and applying antibiotic creams containing neosporin, gramicidin, and bacitracin. In refractory cases the doctor may prescribe the use of antibiotics by mouth, or an injection of penicillin or its derivatives. The condition disappears rapidly with proper therapy.

Herpes simplex, also known as "cold sores," is caused by a viral infection. Herpes simplex can be brought on by any one of a variety of causes. These include excessive exposure to the sun, common colds, the start of menstruation, and intestinal upset. The condition appears as a group of blisters on a reddened base, which later become covered with crusts. If the disorder appears on the lips it is called *herpes buccalis;* on the face, *herpes facialis;* and on the genitals, *herpes progenitalis.*

Treatment of herpes simplex consists of local application of astringent tinctures, antibiotics and, in certain cases, corticosteroid preparations. A more recent experimental treatment is to paint the "herpes" with a neutral red dye, and to follow this with exposure of the affected area to a fluorescent or incandescent light for fifteen minutes. Doctors have successfully used this novel treatment in healing the crusts and blisters, and also in imparting an immunity that causes the herpes to occur less frequently.

Herpes zoster (shingles) is a similar collection of blisters on a reddened base. However, it occurs along the course of a cutaneous nerve, usually on one side of the body; it may, for example, show up first on one side of the forehead and follow the path of the cutaneous nerve down to the eye and nose. This disorder, which appears in older people, is a painful one. If it enters the eye it can impair the cornea, or lens, and may even cause blindness. The causative factor in herpes zoster is a virus related to the one that causes chicken pox. This virus may repose in the body in a dormant fashion, and when it is suddenly irritated this disease results. Sometimes the pain is unbearable and it is necessary for the doctor to prescribe codeine or Demerol to enable the patient to endure it.

Treatment for herpes zoster consists of doses of analgesics, or cortisone, taken orally. Injections of a long-acting cortisone preparation have been used in this condition.

Another common disease of the skin, *pityriasis rosea,* shows up as a rash consisting of irregular-scaling red patches, which cover one fairly large area. This is known as the herald spot, and from it the rash spreads on the body until many irregular areas, from the neck to knee, may be covered with it. Pityriasis rosea is a self-limited disease; it lasts about six to eight weeks and slowly disappears. Treatment consists of the application of mild lotions or creams to soothe the discomfort. Exposure to sunlight or to ultraviolet light may cause the rash to become less conspicuous.

Warts (*verruca*) are irregular, browny growths that may occur in any area of the body. Common warts, the type that appear most frequently, are known as *verruca vulgaris.* Flat warts (*verruca plana*) —despite their name—usually are slightly elevated and are seen in younger people. They occur on the face, hands, feet, or genital tract. The warts that cause the most difficulty occur on the soles of the feet and are known as *plantar warts.*

Warts are caused by special viruses. The best method of treatment is to destroy them by means of acids, electro-desiccation or, occasionally, superficial x-ray.

Eczema of the skin is an inflammation that may appear in a number of different forms. Most commonly it is marked by dry, scaling, reddened areas which appear on the skin. We have discussed contact eczematous dermatitis on pages 151 and 152. Another common eczematous disorder, known as atopic dermatitis, is often seen in allergic patients. It usually attacks infants who develop a scaling condition of the face, neck, and extremities. It can best be treated by using antihistamines internally and corticosteroid creams or liquids externally. Occasionally the creams are covered with clear polyethylene plastic dressings to accelerate absorption of the medication through the skin. Children or adults suffering from atopic dermatitis should avoid eating chocolate, iodized salt, fresh orange juice, or fish products of any kind. Wool clothing and feather pillows must be avoided, and only unscented soaps or cosmetics should be used.

A skin disorder especially prevalent in children is *ringworm* (scientifically called tinea). It can affect the scalp (*tinea capitis*), the body (*tinea corpora*), the groin (*tinea crura*), the nails (*tinea manum*), or the feet (*tinea pedis*). Ringworm is caused by a fungus which can be identified under the microscope or in a properly prepared culture. The infection is characterized by inflammation, redness, and blisters. On the body the lesion takes the shape of a circle, clear in the center and elevated at the periphery, usually with minute blisters.

The treatment for ringworm varies according to the degree of seriousness of the infection. The doctor will prescribe an antifungal cream, powder, spray, or liquid containing fatty acids, salicylic and benzoic acids, Tinaderm® or other proprietary fungicide. If the condition is severe and occurs especially on the scalp and body, the doctor will prescribe antifungal agents such as griseofulvin, to be taken by mouth.

Another skin ailment that shows up occasionally is caused by a form of yeast. Known as *monoliasis,* it is the work of an invader named candida. Monoliasis attacks the nails or appears under the breasts of obese women. Occasionally, it affects the webs of the fingers of women who use large amounts of detergents. Diagnosis is usually made by the doctor, who will prescribe, in milder cases, creams or ointments containing nystatin. In severe cases this drug may be taken orally in tablet form.

19

New Horizons

In May 1972, I was a speaker at the Pilo-Sebaceous Symposium, an international medical congress that met at Crans, Switzerland, to present and discuss new findings in the treatment of the skin and hair. The conference was attended by some five hundred dermatologists, physiologists, physicists, cosmetologists, and microbiologists from many nations. A long list of interesting papers were presented on the management of disorders of the skin and hair. As I listened to these papers and the stimulating discussions that followed them, I could not but be impressed by the energy and dedication with which research into the causes and treatment of these disorders is being pressed forward by devoted researchers. Many of these men and women spend long hours in the laboratory that could otherwise be devoted to their families. I left the conference with the realization that the specialty of dermatology is rapidly becoming one of the most important branches of medicine, in the laboratory as well as in the consulting room and clinic.

Through their continuing investigations, scientists such as these are constantly discovering new facts regarding skin growth and function. They have developed the revolutionary therapies with miracle drugs that we have discussed in this book, such as the use of antibiotics in the treatment of acne, of corticosteroids and methotrexate to alleviate the torments of psoriasis, and the combined therapy of acridine dyes and fluorescent light for herpes simplex. Their work has led to the successful application of corticosteroids for that dangerous and painful disease, herpes zoster; psoralens for sunburn; silicones for wrinkles; and photosensitized hydroquinones for hyperpigmentation. Valuable discoveries in the field of drugs and medicines include the complete sunblocks for use in cases of photoallergy, zinc pyrithione for dandruff, amino acids for the hair, and the new protective emollients. Highly promising experimental work is now being pressed forward in the suggested use of vitamins in high dosages—as, for example, Vitamin E as an antioxidizing agent to prevent aging of the skin—and balanced nutrition for keeping the skin attractive and youthful-looking.

Among other exciting discoveries of hard-working investigators have been the use of antiandrogens to prevent acne, and possibly also in the treatment of pattern baldness, and of steroid anabiolics for possible treatment of that mysterious and stubborn affliction, male pattern baldness. Others have pioneered in the use of laser beams in the treatment of port-wine and other facial marks; ultrasound for warts; cryotherapy, or the use of very low temperatures, in the treatment of malignancies; and the possible use of plastic methylacrylates (which are also effective in cementing fractured bones) in implants for the eradication of wrinkles.

The recent discovery that in atopic dermatitis cases there is a preponderance of IgE antigens may lead to the development of a new therapy for this old, chronic disease. In the area of mental hygiene, new successes have been achieved in treating skin disorders of psychosomatic origin—their symptoms arising from mental or emotional rather than from physical causes—through group psychiatric therapy. Another important advance has been the discovery that many antiseptic chemicals used in cosmetics can cause contact dermatitis. Among these newly detected potential menaces are parabens, hexachlorophene, tribromsalicylanilides (TBS), neomycin, and benzalkonium chloride. It has also been learned that applications of lotions containing isopropyl myristates in spray form can prevent contact dermatitis due to special allergens.

Among other new developments, dermatologists are now performing plastic surgery such as mini-lifts in their consulting rooms. Ozone vapor therapy is being used by beauticians to cleanse the skin, and this promising technique may eventually be adopted by dermatologists.

To be sure, not all innovations prove as successful as one hopes. Today hair transplants are very popular, but in my clinical judgment they have been found unsatisfactory. The hair is not always retained—after four or five years it may be lost entirely—and the procedure is painful and causes scarring. Moreover, the new hair grows in a different pattern and in other directions than the original hair, presenting an unsightly appearance. I do not recommend hair transplants as a beneficial treatment for baldness. I am also opposed to hair weaving and to the practice recently introduced in some quarters of suturing the toupee to the scalp. I have seen too many inflammatory reactions, with continuous pain, resulting after that procedure.

I am an optimist, however, not a pessimist, and I believe in using the new drugs and surveying the unknown horizons for better ways of treating abnormal defects of the skin and improving its functioning. Exciting discoveries are being made at a rate that can only be deeply encouraging, and I am confident that the future will bring forth many new treatments and fresh, unforeseen approaches in the science and art of keeping the skin healthy, young-looking, and beautiful. These findings will originate in the scientist's laboratory and the physician's consulting room, not in the beautician's public relations office.

Appendix I

Common Cosmetics, Irritants, and Allergens*

Ingredients Used in Cosmetics Manufacture Reported to Cause Allergic Reactions

SUBSTANCE	COMMONLY FOUND IN	SYMPTOMS
ACETONE	Nail polish removers	Peeling and splitting of the nails Dermatitis of the fingers, eye areas
ALMOND OIL	Cosmetic creams Lotions Perfumes Soaps	Rhinitis† Dermatitis venenata‡
ALUM	Astringent lotions Anhidrotics	Dermatitis venenata
ALUMINUM ACETATE ALUMINUM CHLORIDE ALUMINUM SULFATE	Astringent lotions Anhidrotics Deodorants	Dermatitis venenata

* Chart courtesy of Ar-Ex Products Co.
† *Rhinitis:* Inflammation of the mucous membrane of the nose
‡ *Dermatitis venenata:* Dermatitis produced by the local action of irritant substances

SUBSTANCE	COMMONLY FOUND IN	SYMPTOMS
AMMONIUM CARBONATE	Permanent wave solutions	Dermatitis of the scalp, forehead, and hands
ANTIMONY COMPOUNDS	Hair dyes	Dermatitis venenata
ARROW ROOT	Dusting powder Dry shampoos	Rhinitis Conjunctivitis
ARSENIC COMPOUNDS	Hair tonics Hair dyes	Dermatitis venenata
BALSAM OF PERU	Perfumes	Dermatitis venenata Rhinitis Perennial hayfever
BARIUM SULFIDE	Depilatories	Dermatitis venenata
BENZALDEHYDE	Cosmetic creams Lotions	Dermatitis venenata
BETANAPHTHOL	Hair dyes Skin peeling preparations	Dermatitis venenata
BISMUTH COMPOUNDS	Bleaching creams Freckle creams	Dermatitis venenata
CALCIUM SULFIDE	Depilatories	Dermatitis venenata
CORNSTARCH	Dusting powders Face powders	Conjunctivitis Rhinitis Perennial hayfever
DIBROM-FLUORESCEIN	Indelible lipsticks	Lip inflammation, often accompanied by respiratory symptoms and dermatitis Gastrointestinal symptoms simulating inflammation of the colon

SUBSTANCE	COMMONLY FOUND IN	SYMPTOMS

GUM ARABIC	Wave sets
	Rouge and powder
	  compacts as a
	  binder
		Atopic coryza*
		Atopic dermatitis
		Gastrointestinal
		  distress
		Asthma

GUM KARAYA	Wave sets
	Toothpaste
	Denture adhesive
	  powder
	Hand lotions
	Rouge and powder
	  compacts as a
	  binder
		Perennial hayfever
		Atopic coryza
		Atopic dermatitis
		Gastrointestinal
		  distress
		Asthma

GUM TRAGACANTH	Wave sets
	Hand lotions
	Rouge and powder
	  compacts as a
	  binder
		Atopic coryza
		Atopic dermatitis
		Gastrointestinal
		  distress
		Asthma

LANOLIN	Cosmetic creams Lotions Shampoos Ointment bases	Dermatitis venenata
LEAD COMPOUNDS	Hair dyes	Dermatitis venenata
LYCOPODIUM	Dusting powders	Rhinitis Perennial hayfever
MERCURY COMPOUNDS	Bleaching creams Freckle creams Hair tonics Medicated soaps	Dermatitis venenata

METHYL HEPTINE CARBONATE	Perfumes
	Toilet waters
	Perfumed cosmetics
		Rhinitis
		Perennial hayfever
		Asthma
		Dermatitis when
		  comes in contact
		  with the skin

* *Atopic coryza:* catarrh of the nasal passages and sinuses, or "cold in the head," with running nose, due to an inherited disposition to allergy to the substance in question

SUBSTANCE	COMMONLY FOUND IN	SYMPTOMS
OILS OF BERGAMOT, CANANGA, CORIANDER, GERANOIL, HELIO-TROPINE, HYDROXY-CITRO-NELLA, LAVENDER, LEMON, LEMONGRASS, LINALOOL, NEROLI, ORANGEPEEL, ORIGANUM, ORRIS, YLANG YLANG	Perfumes Toilet waters Perfumed cosmetics	Inflammation Perennial hayfever Asthma Dermatitis when they come in contact with the skin Photosensitivity
OIL OF CASSIA (CLOVE) OIL OF PEPPERMINT OIL OF SPEARMINT OIL OF WINTERGREEN	Perfumes Toilet waters Perfumed cosmetics Toothpaste Toothpowder	Rhinitis Perennial hayfever Asthma Dermatitis when they come in contact with the skin
OIL OF CITRONELLA	Perfumes Toilet waters Perfumed cosmetics Mosquito repellants	Rhinitis Perennial hayfever Asthma Dermatitis when in contact with skin
ORRIS ROOT POWDER	Toothpaste Dry shampoos Sachets Formerly in most face powders but now only rarely used	Infantile eczema Perennial hayfever Rhinitis Conjunctivitis Asthma

SUBSTANCE	COMMONLY FOUND IN	SYMPTOMS
PARAPHENYL-ENEDIAMINE	Hair dyes Eyebrow and eyelash dyes	Dermatitis venenata
PHENOL	Hand lotions	Dermatitis venenata
POTASSIUM CARBONATE POTASSIUM SULFITE	Permanent wave solutions	Dermatitis of the scalp, forehead, and hands
PYROGALLOL	Hair dyes	Dermatitis venenata
QUININE SULFATE	Hair tonics	Dermatitis venenata
RESORCINOL	Hair tonics	Dermatitis venenata
RICE STARCH	Face powder Dusting powder	Conjunctivitis Rhinitis Perennial hayfever
ROSIN	Hair lacquers	Dermatitis venenata
SALICYLIC ACID	Deodorants Hair tonics	Dermatitis venenata
SODIUM CARBONATE	Permanent wave solutions	Dermatitis of the scalp, forehead, and hands
STRONTIUM SULFIDE	Depilatories	Dermatitis venenata
SULFONAMIDE RESINS	Nail lacquers	Eyelid dermatitis Itching (may be in various locations) Dermatitis venenata
TETRABRAM-FLUORESCEIN	Indelible lipsticks	Lip inflammation, often accompanied by respiratory symptoms and dermatitis Gastrointestinal symptoms simulating colitis

SUBSTANCE	COMMONLY FOUND IN	SYMPTOMS
THIOGLYCOLLIC ACID SALTS	Cold permanent wave preparations	Dermatitis venenata
WHEAT STARCH	Dusting powders Face powders	Conjunctivitis Rhinitis Perennial hayfever
ZINC CHLORIDE ZINC SULFATE	Astringent lotions	Dermatitis venenata

Appendix II

Food Chemistry Chart

The chart that follows contains a list of essential minerals and vitamins, showing the functions of each, and of foods that serve as good sources of each of these vital diet constituents. This chart was prepared by Health Research, of Mokelumne Hill, California, and is reproduced with their permission.

Minerals

Essential Minerals	Functions in Body	Good Sources
Calcium Blood, Bones (W.T.O.)	Necessary for coagulation of the blood, to give firmness and rigidity to bones and teeth, for activating enzymes, for the functions of the muscles, nerves, and heart.	Milk, buttermilk, cheeses, kale, broccoli, celery, cabbage, mustard greens, egg yolk, almonds, Brazil nuts, hazelnuts, whole wheat.
Phosphorus Brain, Bones (T.W.)	Important part of bones, nerves, and brain. Essential in metabolism of fats and carbohydrates, exerts protective effect in blood and muscles.	Dried beans, liver, lean meats, ham, fish, cheese, peanuts, eggs, whole wheat, oatmeal, brown rice.
Iron Blood (O.W.)	Acts as a means of carrying oxygen, needed for tissue respiration, the development of red blood cells, and for normal complexion.	Kidney, tongue, lean beef, liver, clams, oysters, greens, spinach, molasses, wheat germ, bran, egg yolk, chicken, watercress, whole wheat, raisins.

211

Essential Minerals	Functions in Body	Good Sources
Sodium Lymph Blood Tissues (W.T.)	Serves to preserve balance between calcium and potassium to maintain body equilibrium. Acts as a protective agent in blood, aids to prevent excessive loss of water from tissues.	Bananas, butter, bacon, salt, fish, meat stock and broth, crackers, bread, milk, cheese, whole wheat.
Potassium Blood Tissues (W.)	Associated with nitrogen metabolism in the formation and activities of muscle, glandular, nerve, and epithelial tissues. In correct balance, it aids nervous system against irritability.	Dried limas, fish, meat, olives, molasses, prunes, lentils, raisins, almonds, peanuts, spinach, avocados, whole wheat.
Magnesium Bones Muscles (W.T.)	Needed for activation of enzymes, for muscular activity, nerve stability, and bone structure. Involved in elimination of body waste.	Milk, greens, cabbage, carrots, onions, beef, veal, pork, lamb, whole wheat, liver, apples.
Manganese Liver Kidney Pancreas (W.)	Appears essential for growth and reproduction, probably as oxidative catalyst. Necessary for synthesis of Vitamin C in the body.	Barley, beef, dried beans, peas, blueberries, dates, nuts, watercress, rye bread, oatmeal, brown rice, whole wheat.
Sulfur Hair, Nails Bile (O.T.)	Concerned with oxidation processes of the body and represents a part of protein metabolism.	All meats, fish, eggs, milk, dried peas and beans, potatoes, oatmeal, whole wheat.
Silicon Bones Teeth (W.)	Seems necessary in growth of hair, teeth, and nails. Traces found in skeletal structures of the body.	Carrots, green beans, lettuce, cabbage, greens, fresh peas, tomatoes, asparagus, rye, oatmeal, whole wheat.

Essential Minerals	Functions in Body	Good Sources
Chloride Lymph Blood (T.)	Aids digestion, activates enzymes, and is essential to normal gastric secretion. Also, aids in the regulation and stimulation of muscular action.	Oysters, cottage cheese, cauliflower, molasses, milk, macaroni, whole wheat, egg white, watercress.
Copper Liver Spleen (O.T.)	Functions with iron in its transformation into such substances as hemoglobin; aids tissue respiration.	Liver, beans, egg yolk, lobster, shrimp, oatmeal, leafy vegetables, whole wheat.
Iodine Glands (O.)	Essential in the normal regulation of the energy output of the human body and the proper functioning of the thyroid gland. Tends to lessen irritability and nervousness.	Seafoods, and all vegetables grown in soil containing iodine, whole wheat.
Fluoride Blood Bones Teeth (T.)	Decreases incidence of dental caries. Animal experiments show it modifies calcium and phosphorus metabolism. Excess easily toxic.	Milk, egg yolk, oysters, cabbage, mineral water, whole wheat.

NOTE: Exact percentages of mineral losses in food by cooking will vary owing to many varying factors that enter into the process of food preparation. T.—Impaired by high temperature. W.—Dissolved in water. O—Oxidizes.

Vitamins

Vitamins	Mode of Action	Good Sources
A (Fat Soluble) Destroyed by high temperature and oxidation	Promotes growth, appetite, digestion. Important role in connection with eyes, skin, certain respiratory infections, gastrointestinal tract.	Butter, cheese, cream, egg yolks, whole milk, liver, kale, parsley, spinach, carrots, tomatoes, sweet potatoes, fruits, fish liver oil.

Vitamins	*Mode of Action*	*Good Sources*
B$_1$ Thiamin (Water Soluble) Impaired by high temperature	Promotes appetite and tonicity of digestive tract, helps maintain healthy nerves. Important role in neuritis of alcoholism, pregnancy, pellagra, and beri-beri.	Liver, kidney, heart, lean pork, ham, green peas, navy and lima beans, wheat germ, bran, whole wheat, soybeans, baker's and brewer's yeast.
Niacin (Water Soluble) Impair-heat resistant	Has role in certain eye and skin conditions; body swelling in disease; polyneuritis, especially in alcoholism and pregnancy.	Liver, heart, brain, lean meat, eggs, milk, beet greens, spinach, green peas, cauliflower, wheat germ, soybeans, enriched flour, dried yeast.
B$_2$, G. Riboflavin (Water Soluble) Impaired by high temperature	Essential in prevention of pellagra. Has role in certain nervous disturbances, indigestion, nausea, dizziness, insomnia.	Lean meat, especially liver; enriched flour, dry yeasts, milk, and leafy vegetables when consumed in abundance.
C, Ascorbic Acid (Water Soluble) Easily destroyed by heat and oxidation	Increases resistance to infections; prevents scurvy; essential for nutrition of bones, teeth, gums; aids wound healing. Has role in anemic conditions.	Citrus fruits, strawberries, sprouted grains, cabbage (green and raw), cauliflower, dandelion greens, mustard greens, turnip greens, watercress, spinach, peppers, pimentos, parsley, broccoli, brussels sprouts.
D (Fat Soluble) Fairly stable to heat	Regulates utilization of calcium and phosphorus in development of bones and teeth; aids in blood normalization.	Sunshine, fish liver oils, liver, eggs, butter, clams, oysters, salmon, cod, tuna, herring, sardines, leafy vegetables.
E, Tocopherol (Fat Soluble) Withstands fairly high temperature	Anti-sterility vitamin. Has a role in the prevention of miscarriage.	Abundant in cereal grains highest in wheat and corn germ, watercress, lettuce, fresh beef-fat, and glandular organs.

Index

Abrasives, 36, 55
Abscesses, 179
Acetone, 54
Acid mantle, 38, 95, 190
Acids, 188
  and alkali balance, 20, 190
  amino, 102, 203
  aminobenzoic, 95, 101, 119
  ascorbic, 101, 105
  benzoic, 200
  boric, 199
  carbolic, 135
  fatty, 22–23, 200
  folic, 105
  nicotinic, 100–01
  pantothenic, 100, 105
  ribonucleic, 126, 134
  salicylic, 52, 135, 191, 193, 197
  stearic, 163
  tannic, 115
  trichloroacetic, 135
Acne, 14, 46–48, 99, 158, 196
  in girls, 50
  masking of, 77
  oily skin, 52, 54–56
  and the Pill, 51
  scarring, 84
  teenagers, 45
  treatment of, 48–50, 52
Acrolein compound, 157
Adolescence, 46
Advertising, 36, 59, 61, 66, 72–73, 93
After-shave balms, 82–84, 153

Aging, attitude, 25, 59, 122, 126, 130
  and bathing, 35
  skin, 15–16, 76, 126–129, 133–134,
    136, 183, 203
  spots of, 132–133
  in women, 183
Air, 38
  conditioning, 23, 162
  indoor, 42
  pollution, 15, 40, 61, 130, 148,
    156–159
Albinism, variety, 140, 142
Albolene, 40, 130
Albumen, 132
Alcohol, 55, 70
  as antiseptic, 84
  diluted, 54
  rubbing, 78, 199
Alden, H. S., Dr., 152
Alkali and alkalines, 20, 33, 35, 55,
    64, 95, 129, 151, 164, 190
Allantoin complexes, 54, 78, 128,
    160, 193, 197
Allergens, 88–89, 91, 95, 146–148
Allergies, 87, 96, 196
  explosions, 14
  and hypersensitivity, 145–146
  and irritants, 88–90
  lip rouge, 67
  occupational, 149–152
  reactions, 49, 59–62, 145, 159
  skin, 150
  treatment, 154–155, 200

215

Fats, 33, 46, 188
and acids, 22–23, 51, 200
for energy, 99
excess, 19, 190
unsaturated, 22, 104, 129
Feet, soles of, 23, 25, 27, 73, 84, 167–168, 199
Feminine Forever (Wilson), 124, 183
Feminine hygiene sprays, 80
Fibrils, elastic, 126
First Aid, sunburn, 118, 120
Fish, 100, 133, 149
Fog and smog, 117
Follicles, hair, 19, 28, 77, 94, 98–99, 158, 181, 190
Food and Drug Administration, 58, 60, 93, 132, 183
Foods, 100–104, 194
fried, 54
organic, 70, 105, 127
and protein, 102, 133
and purine, 126, 133
spicy, 47
synthetic, 105
Forehead area, 23, 25, 48, 54–55, 73, 119, 159, 163
Formaldehyde resins, 93, 96
Foundation preparations, 40, 54–56, 60, 64, 130, 142, 165
France, 58
Frank, Benjamin, Dr., 125–126, 134
Freckles, 15, 141–144
Freinkel, Ruth K., Dr., 51
Freshener, nonalcoholic, 40–42
Frowns and frowning, 128, 185
Fruit, 49, 71, 100, 127
Fungus, 169, 200

Genetic color scheme, 139
Genital region, 25, 37, 73
Georgetown University Medical Center, 170
Glands, 179, 183
adrenal, 180, 182
apocrine, 23, 25
dysfunction of, 180
eccrine, 23
sebaceous oil, 17, 22–23, 28, 46, 49, 52, 180
and sebum, 179

sex, 47, 50, 125, 179, 186
sweat, 19, 23–25, 28, 38, 180
Glycerin, 33, 64, 95, 191
Goose bumps, 30
Gramicidin, 197
Grime stains, 55, 64, 163

Hair
aids, 43, 82–83, 155, 193–194
brushing, 80
color, 60, 100–101
conditioners, 193
damage, 14, 94
dyes and rinses, 60, 87–91, 151
excess or unwanted, 23, 73, 180–182
follicles, 19, 28, 77, 94, 98–99, 158, 181, 190
growth, 29, 33, 73, 181
length, 14, 49
nutrition, 82, 98
oily, 49
and the Pill, 175–177
and scalp, 84, 180
sprays, 84
straightening, 90–94, 151, 177
teasing of, 177
thinning, 175–176, 181, 189
transplants, 85, 203
Halogenated salicylanides, 90
Halprogin, 200
Hamilton, J. B., Dr., 180–181
Hands, area of, 23, 25, 70, 73
Harvard Medical School, 51
Health products, 59, 167
Heat, 28
rash, 26
systems of, 162–163
summer, 27
Heliophile cult, 113, 120–121
Heparin, 177
Hereditary factor, 31, 89, 115, 139, 141, 148
Herpes simplex, 197–198, 203
Herpes Zoster, 196, 198
Hexachlorophene, 26, 71, 92, 153, 203
Hickey, C., Dr., 190
Hippy minority, 45
Hives, 148

About the Author

DR. IRWIN I. LUBOWE has been practicing medicine for more than forty years. Specializing in dermatology, he conducts a private practice in New York City and serves as Clinical Professor of Dermatology at the New York Medical College and Attending Dermatologist at the New York Metropolitan Hospital Center in New York. Born in New York, he graduated from the College of the City of New York and received his M.D. degree at the same medical college where he now teaches. Noted for his research on the care, hygiene, and treatment of the skin and hair, Dr. Lubowe has contributed many scientific papers on these topics to technical journals. He is author of several books for the general reader, including *New Hope for Your Skin, New Hope for Your Hair,* and *A Teen-Age Guide to Healthy Skin and Hair* (with Barbara Huss). He has also written a scientific text, *Cosmetics and the Skin,* with Fred Wells. Dr. Lubowe served with the Sixty-first Station Hospital in North Africa and Italy during World War II, winning two battle stars. A diplomate of the American Board of Dermatology and Syphilology, he is also a Fellow of the American Academy of Dermatology, the American College of Allergists, the Argentinian Society of Dermatology, and the Royal Society of Health. Dr. Lubowe and his wife have two sons and live in New York City.